MW01673133

THE COMPLETE PEGAN DIET COOKBOOK FOR BEGINNERS

300 Pegan Recipes for your Whole Family to Regain Energy and Feel Fit While Eating Healthy, Prevent Disease, and Enjoy the World of Taste

By
Lisa Calimeris

© Copyright 2022 by LISA CALIMERIS

All rights reserved.

This document provides exact and reliable information regarding the topic and issues covered. The publication is sold with the idea that the publisher is not required to render accounting, officially permitted, or otherwise qualified services. If advice is necessary, legal, or professional, a practiced individual in the profession should be ordered.

Declaration of Principles was accepted and approved equally by a Committee of the American Bar Association and a Committee of Publishers and Associations.

In no way is it legal to reproduce, duplicate, or transmit any part of this document in either electronic means or printed format. Recording of this publication is strictly prohibited, and any storage of this document is not allowed unless with written permission from the publisher. All rights reserved.

The information provided herein is stated to be truthful and consistent, in that any liability, in terms of inattention or otherwise, by any usage or abuse of any policies, processes, or Instructions contained within is the solitary and utter responsibility of the recipient reader. Under no circumstances will any legal responsibility or blame be held against the publisher for any reparation, damages, or monetary loss due to the information herein, either directly or indirectly.

Respective authors own all copyrights not held by the publisher.

The information herein is solely offered for informational purposes and is universal. The presentation of the information is without a contract or any type of guaranteed assurance.

The trademarks that are used are without any consent, and the publication of the trademark is without permission or backing by the trademark owner. All trademarks and brands within this book are for clarifying purposes only and are owned by the owners themselves s, not affiliated with this document.

Table Of Contents

Introduction

In America and increasingly worldwide, the cornerstone of your diet is ultra-processed industrial food produced in ways that threaten the environment, climate, and human health. It's a trend with devastating consequences for humanity and the environment.

Heart disease, diabetes, dementia, cancer, you name it—six out of ten Americans suffer from a chronic condition connected to your ultra-processed food. Around 88 percent of the population is metabolically ill, implying nearly 9 out of 10 have diabetes. It comes at a huge financial cost: Your economy spends one out of every five dollars on health care. And nearly all of it is used to treat chronic illnesses that are almost entirely driven by poor eating habits.

The consequences for the environment are devastating. You've depleted your fresh water sources, destroyed your aquatic and terrestrial ecosystems, and wiped off pollinator, animal, and edible plant species in the cause of generating large swaths of maize, wheat, and soy.

Fossil fuels, water, and soil are the staples of the global economy. Your climate has been greatly destabilized as accc result of this diet.

Our existing food system must be replaced with an ecologically sustainable one that can provide nutritious meals rich in fruits, vegetables, nuts and seeds, legumes, and grass-fed meats.

The way you feed yourselves has consequences for both yourselves and the environment. It is not too late to start repairing this faulty system.

Pegan, a combination of Paleo and Vegan diets, is aimed to address both health and environmental issues. The Pegan diet has all the nutritional advantages of a Paleo diet, but it excludes any animal products.

This diet has several distinct advantages:

Weight loss: This diet is expressly intended to help you lose weight, which is unusual for vegan diets.

Digestive benefits: Your digestive tract will run more smoothly with fewer animal products in your system.

Environmental impact: Animal husbandry has a significant negative influence on your environment and natural resources. Pegan diets restrict the quantity of animal-derived goods consumed.

The Pegan Diet is also good for the environment. Because you consume many fewer animal products in your diet, you do far less environmental harm.

Pegan diet is a notion that has existed for thousands of years.

You'll not only discover the essentials of the Pegan diet in this book, but you'll also find a ton of easy-to-follow recipes that make it simple to tailor the diet to the needs of everyone in the family.

Each day will begin with a breakfast of whole grains or fruit with healthy Fat, followed by lean meat, vegetable, and salad for lunch. Dinner is frequently similar to lunch, with extra salads to keep you full. This book has a wealth of tasty recipes for almost every meal, as well as snacks and sweets that taste wonderful while adhering to your new Pegan diet lifestyle.

This book will teach you all you need to know about the Pegan diet and how to convince your family to follow it. What you'll discover is a low-protein, high-fiber, whole-food plant-based diet that can be customized for everyone from fussy kids who won't eat anything except meatballs to parents who want to instill a healthy lifestyle in their children.

CHAPTER 1:

The Pegan Diet

The Pegan Diet is a popular global diet that arose from a strange blend of Paleo and Vegan diets that made little sense on paper. Dr. Mark Hyman, head of the Cleveland Clinic Centre for Functional Medicine, invented Pegan, claiming that the Pegan style of eating is the most rational and the healthiest diet ever devised for the human race.

The Pegan Diet, created by Dr. Mark Hyman, is a cross between the paleo and vegan diets, based on the idea that paleo and vegan eating (when done properly) value whole, fresh plant foods.

Dr. Hyman has helped numerous men and women all over the globe lose weight, repair their digestive systems, manage difficult disorders like depression and anxiety, and even reverse serious diseases like type 2 diabetes, high blood pressure, and cancer.

To comprehend the convergence, one must first consider the various elements involved:

1.1 The Vegan Diet

A Vegan diet is based on rigorous guidelines, the most important of which is to avoid eating any animal products and prioritize plant-based meals. This diet is deficient in meat and other biomolecule-rich foods such as dairy and eggs. Most vegans are quite picky about what they eat. They avoid processed animal ingredients like gelatin, which is often added to meals, even those that seem vegan, in addition to the limits outlined above.

The result is a minimal diet in calories, cholesterol, and saturated Fat. It is also beneficial to cardiac problems since it helps regulate cholesterol and blood pressure. Veganism is becoming more popular because of its many health advantages.

The vegan diet has several benefits, including lowering the risk of obesity, some malignancies, and type 2 diabetes. However, some amino acids, which are the building blocks of Protein and can only be obtained via nutrition, are lacking in the diet. It also lacks iron, calcium, zinc, and vitamin B12.

1.2 The Paleo Diet

Its adherents were the Stone Age's ancient people. The Paleo diet, like its predecessors, relies only on foods accessible to your forefathers and excludes or limits contemporary foods. The paleo diet emphasizes meat and vegetables, with a little number of fruits and nuts thrown in for good measure. Grains, legumes, added sugar, dairy, and a variety of oils should all be avoided as additions and replacements.

By way of contrast, the cave people, the inventors of the paleo diet, ate grass-fed meat, fish, eggs, nuts, fruit, and organic low-starch vegetables, which your hunter ancestors hunted. Foods including cereals, legumes, refined sugar, potatoes, most dairy products, and some oils are forbidden, despite their fat level is not regulated.

Every meal for most Paleo dieters includes tiny servings of meat. It indicates that meat provides around 30-50 percent of daily energy. Compared to current dietary standards, which suggest that meat should account for 15% to 25% of a day's calories, these amounts are twice as high.

1.3 The "Pegan" Diet

When creating a dietary plan, following a set of principles ensures that you know what to eat and how much to consume. The Pegan diet is simple since the restrictions are considerably more adjustable.

A proper Paleo diet may be too taxing and costly for some people. When you consider the health implications, it's also a concern. On the other hand, veganism is similarly stringent and difficult for individuals to follow. As a result of combining these two opposed diets, the Pegan diet, which offers a great balance of health advantages and minimal restrictions, makes a lot of sense for those of us who wish to live a healthy lifestyle while agreeing to consume a limited amount of animal-based Protein.

The Pegan Diet combines the greatest aspects of veganism with paleo nutrition. Gluten, dairy, soy, maize, potatoes, rice, and sugar are all recommended as foods to avoid. Animal products are seen as an occasional luxury rather than a primary food source on the Pegan Diet, promoting greater eating of vegetables and fruit.

Most diets help you lose weight by restricting your calorie intake and reducing hunger. The Pegan Diet allows you to completely regulate your appetite by eating more nutrient-dense foods like high-quality veggies and lowering total calories via natural caloric reduction or exercise/activity. It has been demonstrated to have a far bigger impact on satiety, helping people feel fuller for longer periods and resist cravings.

The Pegan Diet places a premium on adaptability. Without constraints of tight structures, Pegan may tailor the diet around their lifestyle and vice versa, allowing them to enjoy food as long as it fits within the 13 Pillars of the Pegan Diet. It also means that if you go out to dinner with a buddy, you can still enjoy your meal knowing that you'll be eating lots of fruits and vegetables the following day.

Let's have a look at the 13 pillars of the Pegan diet:

- Sugar should be avoided like the plague. It includes eliminating sugar, wheat, and processed Carbs, which all cause insulin levels to rise. Sugar should be seen as a once-in-a-while treat that you take in moderation in all its forms. It should be regarded as a recreational drug. It's something you do once in a while for fun, but it's not something you consume regularly. Most of your diet is made up of plants. As previously said, vegetables should take up more than half of your plate. The darker the hue, the more intense it is. The more variety there is, the better. Veggies with a high non-starch content should be utilized. Winter squashes and sweet potatoes are OK in moderation (12 cups per day), but don't overdo it! Even though French fries are the most popular vegetable in the United States, they do not qualify.
- Fruit should be avoided. It is where there might be some confusion. Vegan activists suggest consuming all fruit, whereas Paleo followers recommend eating only low-sugar fruits like berries. Most Pegan fans seem to feel better when they stick to low-glycemic foods and regard the remainder as a treat. Berries, kiwis, watermelon, grapes, melons, and other similar fruits should be avoided. Consider dried fruit to be sweets, and only eat it in moderation.
- Pesticides, antibiotics, hormones, and genetically modified organisms (GMOs) should be avoided. Chemicals, preservatives, additives, colors, artificial sweeteners, and potentially dangerous compounds are prohibited. If you don't have an ingredient in your kitchen, you shouldn't eat it.
- Eat foods that are rich in healthy Fat. Omega-3 fatty acids and other beneficial Fat may be found in various foods, including nuts, seeds, olive oil, and avocados, to mention a few. Yes, saturated fat comes from fish, whole eggs, grass-fed or sustainably produced cattle, grass-fed butter, or ghee, as well as organic virgin coconut oil and coconut butter.
- Avoid most vegetable, nut, and seed oils, such as canola, sunflower, maize, grapeseed, and especially soybean oil, which accounts for around 10% of your calories. As for condiments or flavorings, small amounts of expeller or cold-pressed nut and seed oils, such as sesame, macadamia, and walnut, may be utilized. Avocado oil is perfect for high-temperature cooking.
- Dairy should be avoided or consumed in moderation. Dairy isn't beneficial for most people. Therefore, it is recommended to avoid it, except yogurt, kefir, ghee, grass-fed butter, and cheese if you don't like it. Try goat or sheep dairy instead of cow dairy. Also, wherever feasible, pick organic and grass-fed meats.
- Meat and animal products should be served as a side dish, or "Condi-meat," rather than the main course. Meat should be served as a side dish, while vegetables should take center stage. Servings should be no more than 4 to 6 oz each meal. At any one moment, normally cook three or four vegetable side dishes.
- Eat low-mercury seafood that has been raised or harvested responsibly. Sardines, herring, anchovies, and wild-caught salmon are low-mercury and low-toxin options. They should also be collected or grown in an environmentally friendly manner.
- Gluten should be avoided at all costs. Because "Franken wheat" is the most common source of gluten, look for wheat varieties such as einkorn. Wheat should only be ingested on rare occasions if you are not gluten-intolerant. Dr. Alessio Fasano of Harvard, the world's foremost gluten expert, has undertaken research that demonstrates gluten damages the stomach, even in those who aren't gluten-intolerant and exhibit no symptoms.

- Eat gluten-free whole grains in small amounts. They still raise blood sugar levels and can trigger autoimmunity in certain people. Grain can boost blood sugar levels. Low-glycemic grains like black rice, teff, buckwheat, quinoa, and amaranth should be consumed in small amounts (about half a cup per meal). A grain- and bean-free diet may be critical in treating and curing type 2 diabetes, autoimmune illness, and digestive difficulties. • Beans should only be ingested on rare occasions if you're following the 10-Day Detox Diet or a diabetic ketogenic diet. Lentils are the finest legume. Beans that are large and starchy should be avoided. Beans are abundant in fiber, protein, and minerals. However, they may cause digestive problems in certain individuals, and the lectins and phytates in them might obstruct mineral absorption. A high-bean diet may cause blood sugar levels to rise if you have diabetes. Moderate amounts (up to 1 cup per day) are OK.
- Test your plan to make it more personalized. What works well for one person may not work well for another. Experts suggest that everyone eventually work with a properly qualified nutritionist to further personalize their diet via testing.

1.4 The Pegan Pyramid Food

VEGETABLES, HERBS, AND SPICES WITHOUT STARCH: Unlimited, the bottom of the pyramid, comprises colorful, non-starchy vegetables, herbs, and spices. It's better if there's a lot of colors.

According to Mark, anthocyanins, or antioxidants found in blue and purple veggies, may help fight age. Broccoli and artichokes are wonderful examples of green vegetables. As he claims, "Artichokes contain potent detoxifying substances as well as prebiotics, which help to fertilize all your gut's healthy bacteria. Gut microbes are very important for your overall wellness."

Fat That Is Good for You: The doctor recommends three to five servings. While many individuals blame fat for their health concerns, "healthy fat" exists.

You won't eat pasta if you follow the Pegan diet.

"The majority of diets are exclusive. According to the doctor, everything is included in the Pegan food pyramid, emphasizing a quality ".

Protein: up to a cup of lentils and 4 to 6 oz of animal protein

Although the Pegan diet is low in protein, Mark believes that quality animal protein should be included, such as grass-fed beef and dairy products, wild-caught seafood (or sustainably reared if you must eat farmed fish), and pasture-raised meats.

It doesn't have to be expensive, but "you need to know where your food comes from," as Rach puts it.

According to the doctor, the top-notch, dense Protein, and vitamins like B12 found in lean meats and fish are exceedingly difficult to get on a strictly vegetarian diet.

Starchy Veggies and Organic Products: 1/2 cup of drab vegetables, 1 cup of low-glycemic natural product

According to Mark, organic food has a low glycemic index, such as blueberries, raspberries, strawberries, and pomegranates, examples of low glycemic index organic products.

Winter squash and yams are examples of unappealing vegetables that contain beneficial carotenoids and cancer-preventive chemicals.

Grains Without Gluten: ½ to 1 CUP

According to the doctor, you may consume grains but look for "excellent" grains low in starch, low in glycemic index, and low in gluten, such as quinoa and wild rice.

1.5 Sample 14-Day Meal Plan

The four things to remember are:

- Fill your plate with vegetable superstars
- Have 1-2 servings of healthy Fat
- MOST meals should include at least a condiment-sized quantity of protein
- It's best to stay away from inflammatory meals as much as possible (most grains, foods that cause gassiness or constipation, processed and packaged foods).

Day 1	
Breakfast	Cauliflower Fritters with Hummus
Lunch	Brunoise Salad
Dinner	Classic Chicken Cooking with Tomatoes & Tapenade

Day 2	
Breakfast	Overnight Berry Chia Oats
Lunch	Brussels Sprouts and Ricotta Salad
Dinner	BBQ Chicken & Vegetables Sheet Pan

Day 3	
Breakfast	Feta & Quinoa Egg Muffins
Lunch	Celery and Raisins Snack Salad
Dinner	Lamb Burgers

Day 4	
Breakfast	5-Min Heirloom Tomato & Cucumber Toast
Lunch	Dijon Celery Salad
Dinner	Almond-Crusted Swordfish

Day 5	
Breakfast	Greek Yogurt with Walnuts and Honey
Lunch	Fresh Endive Salad
Dinner	Brown Rice Pilaf with Golden Raisins Herb Roasted Chicken

Day 6	
Breakfast	Tahini Pine Nuts Toast
Lunch	Bacon, Brussels Sprout & Spinach Salad
Dinner	Rice and Blueberry Stuffed Sweet Potatoes

Day 7	
Breakfast	Feta - Avocado & Mashed Chickpea Toast
Lunch	Thai Mango Avocado Salad
Dinner	Roasted Pork with Apple-Dijon Sauce

Day 8	
Breakfast	Feta Frittata
Lunch	Grilled Chicken Taco Salad
Dinner	Herbed Lamb Leg

Day 9	
Breakfast	Smoked Salmon and Poached Eggs on Toast
Lunch	Tabbouleh Salad
Dinner	Lemon Caper Chicken

Day 10	
Breakfast	Honey Almond Ricotta Spread with Peaches
Lunch	Caesar Salad
Dinner	Italian Chicken Meatballs

Day 11	
Breakfast	Mediterranean Eggs Cups
Lunch	Greek Potato Salad
Dinner	Orange Roasted Salmon

Day 12	
Breakfast	Low-Carb Baked Eggs with Avocado and Feta
Lunch	Savory Sweet Potatoes
Dinner	Pistachio Sole Fish

Day 13	
Breakfast	Mediterranean Eggs Breakfast Sandwich & Roasted Tomatoes
Lunch	Garlic Crispy Smashed Potatoes
Dinner	Paleo Pizza Crust

Day 14	
Breakfast	Greek Yogurt Pancakes
Lunch	Oven-Roasted Asparagus
Dinner	Wild Rice with Grapes

1.6 Benefit

The Pegan diet focuses on eating healthful, natural foods. It seeks to avoid processed meals and most animal-based items to eat more fruits and vegetables. Because there are no hard and fast rules about what is and isn't acceptable, the emphasis is on making excellent choices within one's lifestyle. Gluten is also avoided in the Pegan diet, a major antioxidant, fiber, vitamins, and minerals.

And it's not just the meals; the Pegan diet is chock-full of vitamins and powders that are supposed to take the place of eating. While many of us are nutritionally inadequate, it is ideal to receive your nutrients via food.

If you're a vegan or vegetarian, there's no denying that this diet allows you to consume a wide range of fruits and vegetables, but it might be difficult to meet your daily protein needs. This diet is deficient in numerous critical elements, including manganese, zinc, vitamin B6, and many more.

Benefits of Pegan Diet:

Manipulation for Better Health - You may eat packaged and processed foods if you want, but they should be avoided for the most part. By eliminating processed foods from one's diet, one's body will become more attuned to its natural balance and will be able to recover from any health problems.

Disease prevention - Diabetes, heart disease, high blood pressure, chronic pain, and dementia may be prevented by concentrating on natural foods and avoiding food additives and preservatives. You can lower your risk of these illnesses and slow down the aging process by concentrating on healthy natural meals.

Weight loss - The Pegan diet allows you to lose weight by eliminating processed and highly processed meals. It is one of its key objectives, and it enables a healthy approach to lose weight without putting in a lot of effort. The emphasis is on choosing healthy choices to reduce weight healthily.

Heart health - The Pegan diet emphasizes natural foods while including a variety of beneficial spices. It encourages you to use more spices in your meals and recipes, good for your heart. Spices including cinnamon, cloves, cumin, nutmeg, and black pepper have been demonstrated to lower blood levels of LDL cholesterol and triglycerides.

Cancer prevention - The Pegan diet has a wide variety of health-promoting foods. It encourages you to eat more veggies, grains, and fruits and add more spices to your diet. Cinnamon, cloves, cumin, nutmeg, and black pepper, among other spices, have lower LDL cholesterol and triglyceride levels in the blood. Cinnamon, cloves, cumin, and black pepper have been found to help prevent cancer by decreasing cancer cell proliferation.

Improving brain function - The Pegan diet improves health by assisting your body in making the most efficient use of its energy. It encourages you to include more spices in your diet, which is beneficial to your brain's performance. Spices like those indicated above have been shown to help with memory and learning.

1.7 10 Tips to Eat Sustainable Food on A Budget

Grow your own

You don't need a nursery, and it takes very little effort to produce a few pots of your favorite spices and veggies, and it's quite satisfying. You may grow on windowsills, patios, and carports, among other places. Start with spices, which might be expensive yet take up very little room.

Try repurposing your empty egg cartons as seedling growers and plant pots made from old bean jars and milk bottles. A single pot of fresh herbs costs about $10 and may last up to three months. Thyme, rosemary, parsley, and basil are among the herbs in the large pots, which come in a range of aromas and smells.

They're simple to grow; keep them in a bright position all year, water them frequently, and trim the leaves as required. You may now get fresh herbs to garnish your meals for a little fee.

Eat less meat

When it comes to buying natural products, meat is at the top of the list. The Soil Association's natural certification ensures that the meat is natural and highly government assistance. Because meat is expensive, but less of it, focus on veggies. When you buy meat, go for the less expensive cuts like shoulder and stomach; they take longer to cook but are often more delicious than the better cuts. Eating less meat is one of the most effective ways to conserve organic food.

Meat contains a lot of saturated fat, which contributes to heart disease and cancer. It is one of the most straightforward methods to eat organic and reduce your carbon footprint. Meat is a high-carbon-intensive food source, so eating less of it will lower your food miles.

Purchasing free-range meat and even organic poultry is a good idea. What you pay for is always what you get. If you purchase the cheapest meat, you're paying for the feed it ate, and it was most likely given cheap junk food.

Reduce waste

The average household wastes 20-30% of their food due to stumbling around the pantry, overbuying, and hopeless hoarding. It is a budget strategy for acquiring higher-quality, natural food. Make sure to start with your best-seasoned meat and veggies and build your meal plan around them. You have an attraction for the oldest vegetables in your refrigerator and toss the fruit into it before cooking.

Buy in bulk

Buying in bulk rather than one item at a time allows one to purchase more. It is more advantageous and cost-effective for you. With less money, you may purchase more food in bulk. You may always keep the remainder of the veggies and fruits in a cold, dry area if needed. You may help the environment by reducing waste since many sellers don't have a clean, cool area to keep surplus veggies and fruits. It will be advantageous to both you and the environment.

Buy seasonal

As you may know, all the finest recipe concepts are based on seasonal ingredients. If you're like the rest of us, you know what to prepare but have no idea what fruits and veggies are in season. You'll go food shopping without thinking about whether the squash or apples will survive long enough for you to eat them. Some applications will inform you what is in season and where you can obtain the freshest produce where you are right now. Fruits and vegetables should be bought frozen.

If you're on a budget, frozen fruits and veggies, particularly out-of-season items like berries in the winter, are a wonderful choice since they're less expensive than fresh food. Waiting till the fruit is on sale will likely be too late.

Cook from scratch

As long as you take care of your fixings and use them sparingly, comfort food varieties are more expensive than cooking raw ingredients from scratch. You prefer to make extra portions of meals that you can eat for lunch the next day or freeze for later use.

Know the 'Clean fifteen.'

The Environmental Working Group has released a list dubbed the 'clean fifteen,' which lists the veggies with the fewest pesticide residues. Avocados, sweet corn, pineapples, cabbage, frozen peas, onions, asparagus, mangoes, papayas, kiwis, eggplant, grapefruit, melon, cauliflower, and yams are the greatest non-natural produce to purchase if you can't tolerate buying all-natural stuff.

Apples, strawberries, grapes, celery, peaches, spinach, sweet chili peppers, imported nectarines, cucumbers, cherry tomatoes, imported snap peas, and potatoes are the foods to avoid.

Join a local organic box scheme

Neighborhood box programs are not always the most cost-effective option; instead, they must battle with the prices of natural grocery store vegetables. They'll provide a good foundation of ingredients for the week, save you time shopping, and support local ranchers. If you're given the option, get a vegetable box without potatoes. It will provide you with a larger selection of fixes. The imported natural product is far more expensive, so stay clear from boxes that include imported stuff. Wherever possible, local food is farmed organically. Because chemicals aren't carried very far, the odds of their being utilized in the soil or sprayed on plants are lower than for other items.

On the other hand, organic foods are not often found close together, or on an island, so you'll have to look for them. Local food is more costly, but it is of higher quality. Buying food from local farms helps the local economy by allowing individuals to spend their money in their community rather than sending it elsewhere.

Create an organic buying group or co-op

Organize a group of people interested in buying organic vegetables and setting up a center. It will increase your buying power since you will have more money to spend. It will also enable you to buy from co-utilizable wholesalers such as Essential-exchanging and Suma center. Communities are a powerful model for business and cooperation that may also help you save money as an individual.

If buying organic is out of the question, make sure the food is pesticide-free by washing it before eating it.

Shop wisely and avoid supermarkets

Natural food is seen as a good thing, yet it may be prohibitively costly as a result. Because general shops are in danger, it is best to avoid them. General stores' prices are frequently available on the internet; write down the prices of the items you frequently purchase and compare them to the prices of online natural products stores, farmers markets, and greengrocers to see who has the best groceries.

CHAPTER 2:

Breakfast Recipes

2.1 Cauliflower Fritters with Hummus

Prep Time: 15 mins

Cook Time: 15 mins

Servings: 4

Ingredients:

- 2 (15 oz) cans chickpeas, divided
- 2 1/2 tbsp olive oil, divided, plus more for frying
- 1 cup onion, chopped, about 1/2 a small onion
- 2 tbsp garlic, minced
- 2 cups cauliflower, cut into small pieces, about 1/2 a large head
- 1/2 tsp salt
- Black pepper
- Topping:
- Hummus, of choice
- Green onion, diced

Directions:

1. Preheat the oven to 400 degrees Fahrenheit. 1 can chickpeas, rinsed and drained, placed on a paper towel to dry completely.
2. Place the chickpeas in a large mixing bowl, discard any loose skins, and toss with 1 tbsp olive oil. Spread the chickpeas on a large baking sheet and season with salt and pepper.
3. Bake for 20 minutes, then toss and bake for another 5-10 minutes, or until crisp.
4. After the chickpeas have been roasted, transfer them to a large food processor and process until they are broken down and crumbled - don't overprocess them and turn them into flour; you want some texture. Fill a small bowl halfway with the mixture and put it aside.
5. Add the remaining 1 1/2 tbsp olive oil to a large pan over medium-high heat. When the pan is hot, add the onion and garlic and sauté for 2 mins, or until the onion and garlic are softly golden brown.
6. After that, add the chopped cauliflower and cook for another 2 mins, or until golden.
7. Reduce to low heat and cover the pan; cook, frequently stirring, until the cauliflower is fork-tender, and the onions are golden brown and caramelized about 3-5 mins.
8. Transfer the cauliflower mixture to a food processor, drain and rinse the remaining can of chickpeas and add them, along with the salt and a touch of pepper, to the food processor.
9. Stop to scrape down the sides as required until the mixture is smooth and begins to ball.
10. Add 1/2 cup roasted chickpea crumbs to the cauliflower mixture in a large mixing bowl and stir until well combined.
11. Pour enough oil into a large mixing bowl over medium heat to lightly coat the bottom of a large pan. Cook the patties in batches until golden brown, approximately 2-3 mins, then turn and cook the other side. Serve.

Nutrition: Calories: 333 Carbs: 45g Fat: 13g Protein: 14g

2.2 Overnight Berry Chia Oats

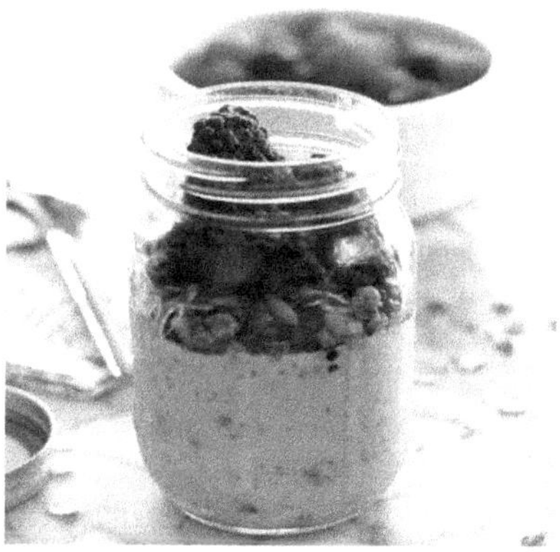

Prep Time: 15 mins

Cook Time: 5 mins

Servings: 1

Ingredients:

- **1/2 c**up Quaker Oats rolled oats

- 1/4 cup chia seeds
- 1 cup milk or water
- Pinch of salt and cinnamon
- Maple syrup, or a different sweetener, to taste
- 1 cup frozen berries of choice or smoothie leftovers
- Toppings:
- Yogurt
- Berries

Directions:

1. Combine the oats, seeds, milk, salt, and cinnamon in a container with a cover and chill overnight. Blend the berries in a blender on the day of serving.
2. Toss the oats with the berry puree, then top with yogurt and additional berries, nuts, honey, or any other garnish you like. Enjoy!

Nutrition: Calories: 405 Carbs: 65g Fat: 11g Protein: 17g

2.3 Feta & Quinoa Egg Muffins

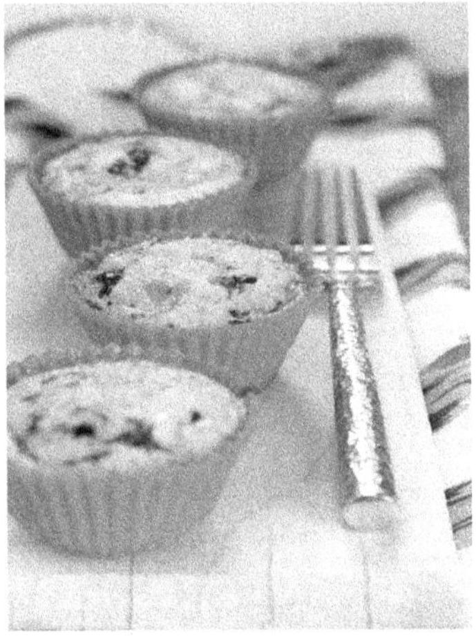

Prep Time: 20 mins

Cook Time: 45-50 mins

Servings: 12

Ingredients:

- 1 cup cooked quinoa
- 2 cups baby spinach, chopped
- ½ cup Kalamata olives
- 1 cup tomatoes
- ½ cup white onion
- 1 tbsp. Fresh oregano
- ½ tsp. Salt
- 2 tsp.+ more for coating pans olive oil
- 8 eggs
- 1 cup crumbled feta cheese
- Also Needed: 12-cup muffin tin

Directions:

1. Preheat your oven to around 350 degrees Fahrenheit. Using a spray of cooking oil, lightly coat the muffin pan cups.
2. Add the oil to a skillet that has been preheated to medium heat. Toss in the onions and cook for two mins once it's heated.
3. Place the tomatoes in a pan and cook for 1 min. Cook, constantly stirring until the spinach leaves have wilted (1 min.).
4. Place the pot on the counter with the oregano and olives in it. Remove it from the equation.
5. Crack the eggs and thoroughly combine them with an immersion stick blender in a mixing dish. Combine the cooked vegetables with the other ingredients.
6. Stir until everything is well blended, then spoon the mixture into prepared muffin cups. Set the timer for 30 mins to bake the muffins until golden brown and firm. Allow for a ten-min cooling period. Serve.

Nutrition: Calories: 295 Carbs: 3g Fat: 23g Protein: 19g

2.4 5-Min Heirloom Tomato & Cucumber Toast

Prep Time: 10 mins

Cook Time: 6-10 mins

Servings: 1

Ingredients:

- 1 small Heirloom tomato
- 1 Persian cucumber
- 1 tsp. Olive oil
- 1 pinch Oregano
- Kosher salt and pepper as desired
- 2 tsp. Low-fat whipped cream cheese
- 2 pieces Trader Joe's Whole Grain Crispbread or your choice
- 1 tsp. Balsamic glaze

Directions:

1. Cut the cucumber and tomato into dice. Except for the cream cheese, combine all ingredients in a mixing bowl. Spread the cheese on the bread and top with the filling. Serve with a drizzle of balsamic glaze on top.

Nutrition: Calories: 239 Carbs: 32g Fat: 11g Protein: 7g

2.5 Greek Yogurt with Walnuts and Honey

Prep Time: 5 Mins

Cook Time: 0 mins

Servings: 4

Ingredients:

- 4 cups Greek yogurt, fat-free, plain, or vanilla
- ½ cup California walnuts, toasted, chopped
- 3 tbsp. Honey or agave nectar
- Fresh fruit, chopped or granola, low-fat (both optional)

Directions:

1. Spoon yogurt into four cups. 2 tbsp walnuts, 2 tbsp honey, 2 tbsp walnuts. Depending on your preference, top with fruit or granola.

Nutrition: Calories 300 Fat: 10g Carbs: 25g Protein: 29g

2.6 Tahini Pine Nuts Toast

Prep Time: 5 mins

Cook Time: 0 mins

Servings: 2

Ingredients:

- 2 whole-wheat bread slices, toasted
- 1 tsp. Water
- 1 tbsp. Tahini paste
- 2 tsp. Feta cheese, crumbled
- Juice of ½ lemon
- 2 tsp. Pine nuts
- A pinch of black pepper

Directions:

1. Combine the tahini, water, and lemon juice in a mixing dish, stir well, and spread over the toasted bread pieces. Serve the remaining ingredients on top of each plate for breakfast.

Nutrition: Calories 142 Fat: 7.6g Carbs: 13.7g Protein: 5.8g

2.7 Feta - Avocado & Mashed Chickpea Toast

Prep Time: 10 mins

Cook Time: 15 mins

Servings: 4

Ingredients:

- 15 oz. Can Chickpeas
- 2 oz. - ½ cup Diced feta cheese
- 1 Pitted avocado
- Fresh juice:
- 2 tsp. Lemon (or 1 tbsp. Orange)
- ½ tsp. Black pepper
- 2 tsp. Honey
- 4 slices Multigrain toast

Directions:

1. Start by toasting the bread. In a colander, drain the chickpeas. Fill the bowl halfway with avocado flesh. Mash them with a large fork/potato masher until the mixture is spreadable.
2. Add the lemon juice, pepper, and feta cheese. Combine the ingredients and distribute them among the four bread pieces. Drizzle honey over the top and serve.

Nutrition: Calories: 337 Carbs: 43g Fat: 13g Protein: 13g

2.8 Feta Frittata

Prep Time: 15 mins

Cook Time: 25 mins

Servings: 2

Ingredients:

- 1 small clove Garlic
- 1 Green onion
- 2 Large eggs
- ½ cup Egg substitute
- 4 tbsp. Crumbled feta cheese - divided
- 1/3 cup Plum tomato
- 4 thin Avocado slices
- 2 tbsp. Reduced-fat sour cream
- Also Needed: 6-inch skillet

Directions:

1. Onion, garlic, and tomato should be thinly sliced or minced. Before slicing the avocado, peel it. Preheat the pan and spray it with cooking oil using the medium temperature option.
2. Combine the egg replacement, eggs, and feta cheese in a mixing bowl. Fill the pan with the egg mixture. Simmer for four to six mins, covered.
3. The remaining feta cheese and tomato should be sprinkled on top. Cover and simmer for another two to three mins, or until the eggs are set.
4. Allow for a five-min cooling period before slicing it in half. Serve with sour cream and avocado.

Nutrition: Calories: 460 Carbs: 8g Fat: 37g Protein: 24g

2.9 Smoked Salmon and Poached Eggs on Toast

Prep Time: 10 mins

Cook Time: 4 mins

Servings: 4

Ingredients:

- 2 oz avocado smashed
- 2 slices of bread toasted
- Pinch of kosher salt and cracked black pepper
- 1/4 tsp freshly squeezed lemon juice
- 2 eggs see notes, poached
- 3,5 oz smoked wild salmon
- 1 TBSP. Thinly sliced scallions
- Splash of Kikkoman soy sauce optional
- Microgreens are optional

Directions:

1. Place the avocado in a small bowl and crush it. Add the lemon juice and a bit of salt to the mixture after that. After that, thoroughly combine everything and put it aside.
2. Poach the eggs and toast the bread for a few mins after that. Once the bread has been toasted, put the avocado on both pieces and then top with smoked salmon on each slice.
3. After that, gently place the poached eggs on top of the toasts. Garnish with scallions and microgreens after adding a splash of Kikkoman soy sauce and cracked pepper.

Nutrition: Calories: 459 Protein: 31 g Fat: 22 g Carbs: 33 g

2.10 Honey Almond Ricotta Spread with Peaches

Prep Time: 5 mins

Cook Time: 8 mins

Servings: 4

Ingredients:

- 1/2 cup Fisher Sliced Almonds
- 1 cup whole milk ricotta
- 1/4 tsp almond extract
- Zest from an orange, optional
- 1 tsp honey
- Hearty whole-grain toast
- English muffin or bagel
- Extra Fisher sliced almonds
- Sliced peaches
- Extra honey for drizzling

Directions:

1. Peaches should be cut into a precise shape and brushed with olive oil. Set it away after that. In a mixing basin, combine the filling ingredients. Remove from the equation.
2. Then just preheat the grill to medium heat. Place the cut side of the peaches on the oiled grill. Close the top and cook until the peaches have softened, around 6-10 mins, depending on the size of the peaches.
3. After that, arrange the peach halves on a serving platter. Fill the hollow with a spoonful of the ricotta mixture (approximately 1 tbsp) (you can also use a small scooper).
4. Slivered almonds, crumbled amaretti biscuits, and honey are sprinkled on top. Mint leaves may be used as a finishing touch.

Nutrition: Calories: 187 Protein: 7 g Fat: 9 g Carbs: 18 g

2.11 Mediterranean Eggs Cups

Prep Time: 10 mins

Cook Time: 20 mins

Servings: 8

Ingredients:

- 1 cup spinach, finely diced
- 1/2 yellow onion, finely diced
- 1/2 cup sliced sun-dried tomatoes
- 4 large basil leaves, finely diced
- Pepper and salt to taste
- 1/3 cup feta cheese crumbles
- 8 large eggs
- 1/4 cup milk (any kind)

Directions:

1. Preheat the oven to 375 degrees Fahrenheit. The dough sheet should then be rolled into a 12x8-inch rectangle. Then, lengthwise, split it in two.
2. After that, cut each half crosswise into four pieces, resulting in eight (4x3-inch) pieces of dough. Then push each into the bottom and up the muffin cup's edges that haven't been oiled.
3. If necessary, trim the dough to avoid it from touching. Remove from the equation. Then, whisk the eggs, salt, and pepper until well combined in a mixing dish. Remove from the equation.
4. In a 12-inch skillet, melt the butter over medium heat until it sizzles, then add the bell peppers. You'll need to cook it for 2-3

mins, stirring periodically, or until crisply tender.

5. After that, add the spinach leaves and simmer until they are wilted. After that, just add the egg mixture and prosciutto.
6. Divide the mixture equally among the muffin cups that have been prepared. Finally, bake for 14-17 mins, or until golden brown on top.

Nutrition: Calories: 240 Protein: 9 g Fat: 16 g Carbs: 13 g

2.12 Low-Carb Baked Eggs with Avocado and Feta

Prep Time: 10 mins

Cook Time: 15 mins

Servings: 2

Ingredients:

- 1 avocado
- 4 eggs
- 2-3 tbsp. Crumbled feta cheese
- Nonstick cooking spray
- Pepper and salt to taste

Directions:

1. At begin, preheat the oven to 400 degrees Fahrenheit. After the oven has reached the desired temperature, place the gratin plates directly on the baking sheet.
2. After that, cook the dishes in the oven for approximately 10 mins. Following that, you must break the eggs into separate ramekins.
3. Allow for at least 10 mins for the avocado and eggs to get to room temperature. Then, thoroughly peel the avocado and cut each half into 6-8 pieces.
4. Remove the plates from the oven and coat them with non-stick cooking spray. After that, place all the sliced avocados in the bowls and crack two eggs into each. Serve with feta cheese, pepper, and salt to taste.

Nutrition: Calories: 280 Protein: 11 g Fat: 23 g Carbs: 10 g

2.13 Mediterranean Eggs Breakfast Sandwich & Roasted Tomatoes

Prep Time: 15 mins

Cook Time: 10 mins

Servings: 2

Ingredients:

- Salt & pepper
- ¼ cup of egg whites
- 1 tsp fresh herbs chopped
- 1 ciabatta roll seeded whole grain
- 1 tsp butter
- 1-2 slices Muenster cheese
- 1 tbsp pesto
- About ½ cup roasted tomatoes
- 10 oz' grape tomatoes
- 1 tbsp extra-virgin olive oil
- Black pepper and salt to taste

Directions:

1. The butter must first be melted in a small nonstick pan over medium heat. The egg whites should next be mixed with pepper and salt.
2. After that, top it with fresh herbs. Cook for another 3-4 mins or until the eggs are done, then gently turn it.
3. Toast the ciabatta bread in the toaster in the meanwhile. Place the egg on the bottom half of the sandwich buns, then cover with cheese.
4. Add the top half of the roll and the roasted tomatoes. Preheat the oven to 400 degrees Fahrenheit for the roasted tomato. The tomatoes should then be cut in half lengthwise.
5. Drizzle with olive oil and place on a baking pan. Roast it in the oven for approximately 20 mins after seasoning it with pepper and salt. When finished, the skin will seem wrinkled.

Nutrition: Calories: 458 Protein: 21 g Fat: 24 g Carbs: 51 g

2.14 Greek Yogurt Pancakes

Prep Time: 10 mins

Cook Time: 5 mins

Servings: 2

Ingredients:

- 1 cup all-purpose flour
- 1 cup whole-wheat flour
- 1/4 tsp salt
- 4 tsp baking powder
- 1 tbsp sugar
- 1 1/2 cups unsweetened almond milk
- 2 tsp vanilla extract
- 2 large eggs
- 1/2 cup plain 2% Greek yogurt
- Fruit, for serving
- Maple syrup, for serving

Directions:

1. To begin, place the curds into a mixing basin and whisk them thoroughly until

creamy. After that, you'll need to add the egg whites and whisk them well until they're all incorporated.

2. Then, in a separate dish, combine the wet and dry ingredients. To blend, stir everything together. It will be a very thick batter.
3. The batter is then spooned into a sprayed medium-high-heat pan. The batter should yield four big pancakes.
4. When the pancakes start to bubble a little on the surface, you'll have to turn them once more. Cook until both sides are golden brown.

Nutrition: Calories: 166 Protein: 14 g Fat: 5 g Carbs: 52g

2.15 Mediterranean Feta and Quinoa Egg Muffins

Prep Time: 15 mins

Cook Time: 15 mins

Servings: 12

Ingredients:

- 2 cups baby spinach finely chopped
- 1 cup chopped or sliced cherry tomatoes
- 1/2 cup finely chopped onion
- 1 tbsp chopped fresh oregano
- 1 cup crumbled feta cheese
- 1/2 cup chopped {pitted} kalamata olives
- 2 tsp vegetable oil
- 1 cup cooked quinoa
- 8 eggs
- 1/4 tsp salt

Directions:

1. Preheat your oven to around 350 degrees Fahrenheit, line a baking sheet with 12 silicone muffin holders, coat a 12-cup muffin tray with oil, and put it aside.
2. Heat the skillet to medium and finely chop the veggies. After that, add the onion and vegetable oil and cook for 2 mins.
3. Then add the tomatoes and cook for another min, then add the spinach and cook for another min, or until wilted.
4. Place the beaten egg in a mixing bowl, then add a variety of veggies, such as feta cheese, quinoa, and the veggie combination, as well as salt, and stir well until everything is thoroughly incorporated.
5. Pour the prepared batter into oiled muffin pans or silicone cups, evenly dividing the batter. Then bake it for around 30 mins in the oven.

Nutrition: Calories: 113 Protein: 6 g Fat: 7 g Carbs: 5 g

2.16 Mediterranean Eggs

Prep Time: 15 mins

Cook Time: 20 mins

Servings: 2

Ingredients:

- 5 tbsp. Of divided olive oil
- 2 diced medium-sized Spanish onions
- 2 diced red bell peppers
- 2 minced cloves garlic
- 1 tsp cumin seeds
- 4 diced large ripe tomatoes
- 1 tbsp of honey
- Salt
- Freshly ground black pepper
- 1/3 cup crumbled feta
- 4 eggs
- 1 tsp zaatar spice
- Grilled pita during serving

Directions:

1. 3 tbsp olive oil, heated in a skillet over medium heat Sauté the cumin seeds, onions, garlic, and red pepper for a few mins in the oil.
2. After that, add the chopped tomatoes and season to taste with salt and pepper and simmer for approximately 10 mins, or until they mix and make a light sauce.
3. That means half of the work is already done. Now all you must do is crack the eggs into the sauce and poach them.
4. However, you must remember to boil the egg whites while leaving the yolks runny. It takes roughly 8 to 10 mins to do this task.
5. Add some feta and olive oil with zaatar spice to the plate to round out the taste. Serve with grilled pita bread.

Nutrition: Calories: 304 Protein: 12 g Fat: 16 g Carbs: 28 g

2.17 Pastry-Less Spanakopita

Prep Time: 5 mins

Cook Time: 20 mins

Servings: 4

Ingredients:

- 1/8 tsp black pepper, add as per taste
- 1/3 cup of Extra virgin olive oil
- 4 lightly beaten eggs

- 7 cups of Lettuce, preferably a spring mix (mesclun)
- 1/2 cup of crumbled Feta cheese
- 1/8 tsp of Sea salt, add to taste
- 1 finely chopped medium yellow onion

Directions:

1. Preheat the oven at 180 degrees Celsius and oil the flan dish. Once the onions are transparent, pour the extra virgin olive oil into a big saucepan and cook it over medium heat with them.
2. Stir in the greens until all the ingredients have wilted. Season the greens with salt and pepper, then transfer them to the prepared dish and top with feta cheese.
3. Pour in the eggs and bake for 20 mins, or until it is well cooked and slightly browned.

Nutrition: Calories: 325 Protein: 11.2 g Fat: 27.9 g Carbs: 7.3 g

2.18 Date and Walnut Overnight Oats

Prep Time: 5 mins

Cook Time: 20 mins

Servings: 2

Ingredients:

- ¼ Cup Greek Yogurt, Plain
- 1/3 cup of yogurt - 2/3 cup of oats
- 1 cup of milk
- 2 tsp date syrup or you can also use maple syrup or honey - 1 mashed banana
- ¼ tsp cinnamon
- ¼ cup walnuts
- Pinch of salt (approx.1/8 tsp)

Directions:

1. First, combine all ingredients in a mason jar or a small dish. After that, thoroughly whisk and combine all the ingredients. Refrigerate it overnight after carefully covering it.
2. The following morning, take it out, add additional liquid or cinnamon if necessary, and serve cold. (However, you may microwave it for those with a hotter palette.)

Nutrition: Calories: 350 Protein: 14 g Fat: 12 g Carbs: 49 g

2.19 Pear and Mango Smoothie

Prep Time: 5 mins

Cook Time: 0 mins

Servings: 1

Ingredients:

- 1 cored & chopped ripe mango
- ½ pitted & chopped mango, peeled
- 1 cup chopped kale
- ½ cup Greek yogurt plain
- 2 cubes ice

Directions:

1. Puree the pear, mango, yogurt, kale, & mango in a blender. Blend in the ice until it forms a smooth texture. Serve and have fun!

Nutrition: Calories: 293, Fat: 8 g Carbs: 53 g Protein: 8g

2.20 Eggplant Salad

Prep Time: 20 mins

Cook Time: 15 mins

Servings: 8

Ingredients:

- 1 large eggplant, washed and cubed
- 1 tomato, seeded and chopped
- 1 small onion, diced
- 2 tbsp parsley, chopped
- 2 tbsp extra virgin olive oil
- 2 tbsp distilled white vinegar
- ½ cup feta cheese, crumbled
- Salt as needed

Directions:

1. Preheat the grill to medium-high heat. Using a knife or fork, pierce the eggplant a few times. Grill the eggplants for approximately 15 mins, or until they're browned.
2. Place it on the side and set it aside to cool. Remove the eggplant's peel and dice the pulp. Add the parsley, onion, tomato, olive oil, feta cheese, and vinegar to the pulp in a mixing bowl.
3. Combine all ingredients in a mixing bowl and refrigerate for 1 hour. Enjoy with a pinch of salt!

Nutrition: Calories: 99 Fat: 7g Carbs: 7g Protein: 3.4g

2.21 Artichoke Frittata

Prep Time: 5 mins

Cook Time: 10 mins

Servings: 4

Ingredients:

- 8 large eggs
- ¼ cup Asiago cheese, grated
- 1 tbsp fresh basil, chopped

- 1 tsp fresh oregano, chopped
- Pinch of salt
- 1 tsp extra virgin olive oil
- 1 tsp garlic, minced
- 1 cup canned artichokes, drained
- 1 tomato, chopped

Directions:

1. Preheat the oven to broil mode. Whisk the eggs, Asiago cheese, oregano, basil, salt, and pepper in a medium mixing bowl. In a mixing dish, combine all the ingredients.
2. Add olive oil to a large ovenproof skillet and heat over medium-high heat. Sauté for 1 min after adding the garlic. Remove the skillet from the heat and add the egg mixture.
3. Return the pan to heat and top the eggs with artichoke hearts and tomato. Cook for 8 mins without disturbing the frittata.
4. Broil the skillet for 1 min, or until the top is gently browned. Serve the frittata in four slices. Enjoy!

Nutrition: Calories: 199 Fat: 13g Carbs: 5g Protein: 16g

2.22 Full Eggs in a Squash

Prep Time: 15 mins

Cook Time: 20 mins

Servings: 5

Ingredients:

- 2 acorn squash
- 6 whole eggs
- 2 tbsp extra virgin olive oil
- Salt and pepper as needed
- 5-6 pitted dates
- 8 walnut halves
- A fresh bunch of parsley

Directions:

1. Preheat the oven to 375 degrees Fahrenheit (190 degrees Celsius). Prepare 3 slices with holes by slicing the squash crosswise. When slicing the squash, make sure each slice measures 34 inches in thickness.
2. Take the seeds out of the slices. Preheat your oven to around 350°F and prepare a baking sheet with parchment paper. Season the slices with salt and pepper and place them on the baking sheet.
3. Preheat the oven to 200°F and bake for 20 mins. On a cutting board, chop the walnuts and dates. Remove the baking dish from the oven and sprinkle olive oil over the pieces.
4. Season with pepper and salt and crack an egg into each of the holes in the slices. Top with walnuts that have been chopped. Cook for another 10 mins. Add maple syrup and parsley to finish.

Nutrition: Calories: 198 Fat: 12g Carbs: 17g Protein: 8g

2.23 Barley Porridge

Prep Time: 5 mins

Cook Time: 25 mins

Servings: 4

Ingredients:

- 1 cup barley
- 1 cup wheat berries
- 2 cups unsweetened almond milk
- 2 cups water
- ½ cup blueberries
- ½ cup pomegranate seeds
- ½ cup hazelnuts, toasted and chopped
- ¼ cup honey

Directions:

1. Fill a medium saucepan halfway with water and set it over medium-high heat. Bring the water, barley, almond milk, wheat berries, and barley to a boil. Reduce the heat to low and continue to cook for another 25 mins.
2. 2 tbsp blueberries, 2 tbsp pomegranate seeds, 2 tbsp hazelnuts, and 1 tbsp honey, divided among serving dishes. Serve and have fun!

Nutrition: Calories: 295 Fat: 8g Carbs: 56g Protein: 6g

2.24 Tomato and Dill Frittata

Prep Time: 5 mins

Cook Time: 10 mins

Servings: 4

Ingredients:

- 2 tbsp olive oil
- 1 medium onion, chopped
- 1 tsp garlic, minced
- 2 medium tomatoes, chopped
- 6 large eggs
- ½ cup half and half
- ½ cup feta cheese, crumbled
- ¼ cup dill weed
- Salt as needed
- Ground black pepper as needed

Directions:

1. Preheat the oven to 400 degrees Fahrenheit (200 degrees Celsius). Heat the olive oil in a large ovenproof skillet over medium-high heat. Stir in the onion, garlic, and tomatoes and cook for 4 mins.
2. While they're cooking, whisk together your eggs, half-and-half cream, and season with pepper and salt in a mixing dish.
3. Pour the mixture into the pan with the veggies, then top with feta cheese crumbles and dill weed. Allow it to cook for 3 mins with the lid on.
4. Preheat your oven to around 350°F and bake the pan for 10 mins. Serve immediately.

Nutrition: Calories: 191 Fat: 15g Carbs: 6g Protein: 9g

2.25 Strawberry and Rhubarb Smoothie

Prep Time: 5 mins

Cook Time: 3 mins

Servings: 1

Ingredients:

- 1 rhubarb stalk, chopped
- 1 cup fresh strawberries, sliced
- ½ cup plain Greek strawberries
- Pinch of ground cinnamon
- 3 ice cubes

Directions:

1. Fill a small saucepan halfway with water and set it over high heat. Bring to a boil, then add the rhubarb and cook for another 3 mins. Drain and puree in a blender.
2. Pulse the strawberries, honey, yogurt, and cinnamon together until smooth. Blend in the ice cubes until the mixture is thick and lump-free. Pour into a chilled glass and enjoy.

Nutrition: Calories: 295 Fat: 8g Carbs: 56g Protein: 6g

2.26 Bacon and Brie Omelet Wedges

Prep Time: 10 mins

Cook Time: 10 mins

Servings: 6

Ingredients:

- 2 tbsp olive oil
- 7 oz smoked bacon
- 6 beaten eggs
- Small bunch chives, snipped
- 3 ½ oz brie, sliced
- 1 tsp red wine vinegar
- 1 tsp Dijon mustard
- 1 cucumber, halved, deseeded, and sliced diagonally
- 7 oz' radish, quartered

Directions:

1. Set your grill to high and turn it on. Place 1 tsp of oil in a small saucepan and heat up. Fry the lardons until they are crisp. Using kitchen paper, drain the lardon.
2. Place a nonstick cast iron frying pan over the grill and heat 2 tbsp of oil. Combine the lardons, eggs, chives, and ground pepper in a frying pan. Cook on low until they're almost done.
3. Place the brie on top and cook until it is set and golden in color. Cut it into wedges after removing it from the pan.
4. Mix olive oil, mustard, vinegar, and seasoning in a small dish to make the dressing. Mix in the cucumber and serve with the omelet wedges.

Nutrition: Calories: 35 Fat: 31g Carbs: 3g Protein: 25g

2.27 Pearl Couscous Salad

Prep Time: 15 mins

Cook Time: 0 mins

Servings: 6

Ingredients:

- For Lemon Dill Vinaigrette:
- Juice of 1 large-sized lemon
- 1/3 cup of extra virgin olive oil
- 1 tsp of dill weed
- 1 tsp of garlic powder
- Salt as needed
- Pepper
- For Israeli Couscous:
- 2 cups of Pearl Couscous
- Extra virgin olive oil
- 2 cups of halved grape tomatoes
- Water as needed
- 1/3 cup of finely chopped red onions
- ½ of a finely chopped English cucumber
- 15 oz of chickpeas
- 14 oz of artichoke hearts (roughly chopped up)
- ½ cup of pitted Kalamata olives
- 15-20 pieces of fresh basil leaves, roughly torn and chopped up
- 3 oz of fresh baby mozzarella

Directions:

1. Combine all the ingredients mentioned under the vinaigrette in a mixing bowl to make the vinaigrette. Combine all the ingredients in a large mixing bowl and set aside. Place a medium-sized heavy pot over medium-high heat.
2. Allow 2 tbsp of olive oil to heat up in the pan. Cook until the couscous is golden brown, then add it. According to the package Directions, cook the couscous using 3 cups of boiling water.
3. Drain in a colander and set aside when finished. Add the other ingredients to a large mixing bowl, except the cheese and basil.
4. Mix in the cooked couscous and basil until everything is thoroughly combined. Stir the vinaigrette well before adding it to the couscous salad. Mix thoroughly.
5. As needed, adjust the seasoning. Toss in the mozzarella cheese. Serve with basil as a garnish. Enjoy!

Nutrition: Calories: 393 Fat: 13g Carbs: 57g Protein: 13g

2.28 Coconut Porridge

Prep Time: 15 mins

Cook Time: 0 mins

Servings: 6

Ingredients:

- Powdered erythritol as needed
- 1 ½ cups almond milk, unsweetened
- 2 tbsp vanilla protein powder
- 3 tbsp Golden Flaxseed meal
- 2 tbsp coconut flour

Directions:

1. Combine a mixing dish with a flaxseed meal, protein powder, and coconut flour. Pour the mixture into the pot (placed over medium heat).
2. Stir in the almond milk and let aside to thicken. Serve with the preferred quantity of sweetener. Enjoy!

Nutrition: Calories: 259 Fat: 13g Carbs: 5g Protein: 16g

2.29 Crumbled Feta and Scallions

Prep Time: 5 mins

Cook Time: 15 mins

Servings: 12

Ingredients:

- 2 tbsp of unsalted butter
- ½ cup of chopped up scallions
- 1 cup of crumbled feta cheese
- 8 large-sized eggs
- 2/3 cup of milk
- ½ tsp of dried Italian seasoning
- Salt as needed
- Freshly ground black pepper as needed
- Cooking oil spray

Directions:

1. Preheat the oven to 400 degrees Fahrenheit (200 degrees Celsius). Grease a 3- to 4-oz muffin tray with frying oil. Preheat a nonstick skillet over medium heat.
2. Allow the butter to soften before adding it. Stir in half of the scallions and cook for another min. Keeping them to the side is a good idea. Whisk the eggs, Italian spice, and milk in a medium-sized mixing bowl.
3. Mix in the feta cheese and stir-fried scallions. Season with salt and pepper. Fill the muffin tray halfway with the batter. Bake for 15 mins with the muffin tray in the oven. With a sprinkling of scallions on top, serve.

Nutrition: Calories: 106 Fat: 8g Carbs: 2g Protein: 7g

2.30 Quinoa Chicken Salad

Prep Time: 15 mins

Cook Time: 20 mins

Servings: 8

Ingredients:

- 2 cups of water
- 2 cubes of chicken bouillon
- 1 smashed garlic clove
- 1 cup of uncooked quinoa
- 2 large-sized chicken breasts cut up into bite-sized portions and cooked
- 1 large-sized diced red onion
- 1 large-sized green bell pepper
- ½ cup of Kalamata olives
- ½ cup of crumbled feta cheese
- ¼ cup of chopped up parsley
- ¼ cup of chopped up fresh chives
- ½ tsp of salt
- 1 tbsp of balsamic vinegar
- ¼ cup of olive oil

Directions:

1. Bring your water, garlic, and bouillon cubes to a boil in a saucepan. Reduce the heat to medium-low and stir in the quinoa.

2. Simmer for 15-20 mins, or until the quinoa is soft and has absorbed all the liquid. Scrape the quinoa into a large mixing basin, discarding the garlic cloves.
3. Combine the cooked chicken breast, bell pepper, onion, feta cheese, chives, salt, and parsley in a small bowl.
4. Lemon juice, olive oil, and balsamic vinegar are drizzled on top. Stir everything together until it's well combined. Warm it up and enjoy it!

Nutrition: Calories: 99 Fat: 7g Carbs: 7g Protein: 3.4g

2.31 Spicy Early Morning Seafood Risotto

Prep Time: 5 mins

Cook Time: 15 mins

Servings: 4

Ingredients:

- 3 cups of clam juice
- 2 cups of water
- 2 tbsp of olive oil
- 1 medium-sized chopped up onion
- 2 minced cloves of garlic
- 1 ½ cups of Arborio Rice
- ½ cup of dry white wine
- 1 tsp of Saffron
- ½ tsp of ground cumin
- ½ tsp of paprika
- 1 pound of marinara seafood mix
- Salt as needed
- Ground pepper as needed

Directions:

1. Put the clam juice and water in a pot over high heat and bring the mixture to a boil. Turn off the heat.
2. In a heavy-bottomed saucepan, cook the garlic and onion in oil over medium heat until a pleasant aroma emerges.
3. Stir in the rice for another 2-3 mins, or until the rice is well coated in oil. Pour in the wine, followed by the saffron.
4. Stir continually until all the liquid has been absorbed. 1 cup at a time, add the cumin, clam juice, and paprika combination, stirring well after each addition.
5. Cook the rice for 20 mins, or until it is perfectly cooked. Cook for another 5-7 mins after adding the seafood marinara mix.
6. Season with a pinch of salt and pepper. Place the entrée on a serving platter. Serve immediately.

Nutrition: Calories: 386 Fat: 7g Carbs: 55g Protein: 21g

2.32 Rocket Tomatoes and Mushroom Frittata

Prep Time: 5 mins

Cook Time: 15 mins

Servings: 4

Ingredients:

- 2 tbsp of butter
- 1 chopped up medium-sized onion
- 2 minced cloves of garlic
- 1 cup of coarsely chopped baby rocket tomato
- 1 cup of sliced button mushrooms
- 6 large pieces of eggs
- ½ cup of skim milk
- 1 tsp of dried rosemary
- Salt as needed
- Ground black pepper as needed

Directions:

1. Preheat the oven to 400 degrees Fahrenheit (200 degrees Celsius). Place a large oven-safe pan over medium-high heat. Preheat the oil.
2. For around 2 mins, stir fry your garlic and onion. Cook for 3 mins after adding the mushroom, rosemary, and rockets. In a medium-sized mixing basin, whisk together the eggs and milk.
3. Add a little salt and pepper to taste. Pour the egg mixture over the veggies in the pan.
4. Reduce to a low heat setting and cover with a lid. Allow 3 mins for it to cook. Place the pan in the oven and bake for 10 mins, or until it is completely set.
5. Reduce to a low heat setting and cover with a lid. Allow 3 mins for it to cook. Bake for another 10 mins after transferring the pan to the oven. Serve immediately.

Nutrition: Calories: 189 Fat: 13g Carbs: 6g Protein: 12g

2.33 Cheesy Olives Bread

Prep Time: 1 hour and 40 mins

Cook Time: 30 mins

Servings: 10

Ingredients:

- 4 cups whole-wheat flour

- 3 tbsp. Oregano, chopped
- 2 tsp. Dry yeast
- ¼ cup olive oil
- 1 ½ cups black olives, pitted and sliced
- 1 cup of water
- ½ cup feta cheese, crumbled

Directions:

1. Combine the flour, water, yeast, and oil in a mixing basin. Make sure to thoroughly mix and knead your dough. Place the dough in a basin, cover with plastic wrap, and let aside for 1 hour to rise.
2. Divide the dough into two basins and stretch each ball out as far as possible. Fill each ball with the remaining ingredients and tuck them inside. Re-knead the dough well.
3. Flatten the balls slightly and set them aside for another 40 mins. Place the balls on a baking sheet lined with parchment paper, slit each one, and bake for 30 mins at 425F.
4. As a Mediterranean breakfast, serve the bread.

Nutrition: Calories 251 Fat: 7.3g Carbs: 39.7g Protein: 6.7g

2.34 Sweet Potato Tart

Prep Time: 10 mins

Cook Time: 1 hour and 10 mins

Servings: 8

Ingredients:

- 2 pounds' sweet potatoes, peeled and cubed
- ¼ cup olive oil + a drizzle
- 7 oz. Feta cheese, crumbled
- 1 yellow onion, chopped
- 2 eggs, whisked
- ¼ cup almond milk
- 1 tbsp. Herbs de Provence
- A pinch of salt and black pepper
- 6 phyllo sheets

Directions:

1. Toss the potatoes with half of the oil, salt, and pepper in a mixing bowl then lay out on a baking sheet fitted with parchment paper and roast for 25 mins at 400F.
2. Meanwhile, heat half of the remaining oil in a skillet over medium heat, add the onion, and cook for 5 minutes.
3. Toss the eggs with the milk, feta, herbs, salt, pepper, onion, sweet potatoes, and the remaining oil in a mixing bowl.
4. Arrange the phyllo sheets in a tart pan and sprinkle a little oil over them. Spread the sweet potato mixture evenly in the pan.
5. Preheat oven to 350°F and bake for 20 mins, covered with tin foil. Remove the tin foil and bake the pie for another 20 mins. Cool completely before slicing and serving for breakfast.

Nutrition: Calories 476 Fat: 16.8g Carbs: 68.8g Protein: 13.9g

2.35 Stuffed Pita Breads

Prep Time: 5 mins

Cook Time: 15 mins

Servings: 4

Ingredients:

- 1 ½ tbsp olive oil
- 1 tomato, cubed
- 1 garlic clove, minced
- 1 red onion, chopped
- ¼ cup parsley, chopped
- 15 oz. Canned fava beans, drained and rinsed
- ¼ cup lemon juice
- Salt and black pepper to the taste
- 4 whole-wheat pita bread pockets

Directions:

1. Over medium heat, heat the oil in a skillet, add the onion, swirl, and cook for 5 mins. Stir in the other ingredients and simmer for another 10 mins.
2. Serve the pita pockets stuffed with this mixture for breakfast.

Nutrition: Calories 382 Fat: 1.8g Carbs: 66g Protein: 28.5g

2.36 Blueberries Quinoa

Prep Time: 5 mins

Cook Time: 0 mins

Servings: 4

Ingredients:

- 2 cups almond milk
- 2 cups quinoa, already cooked
- ½ tsp cinnamon powder
- 1 tbsp. Honey - 1 cup blueberries
- ¼ cup walnuts, chopped

Directions:

1. Toss the quinoa with the milk and the other ingredients in a mixing bowl, divide into smaller bowls, and serve breakfast.

Nutrition: Calories 284 Fat: 14.3g Carbs: 15.4g Protein: 4.4g

2.37 Endives, Fennel and Orange Salad

Prep Time: 5 mins

Cook Time: 0 mins

Servings: 4

Ingredients:

- 1 tbsp. Balsamic vinegar
- 2 garlic cloves, minced
- 1 tsp. Dijon mustard
- 2 tbsp. Olive oil
- 1 tbsp. Lemon juice
- Sea salt and black pepper to taste
- ½ cup black olives, pitted and chopped
- 1 tbsp. Parsley, chopped
- 7 cups baby spinach
- 2 endives, shredded
- 3 medium navel oranges, peeled and cut into segments
- 2 bulbs fennel, shredded

Directions:

1. Combine the spinach, endives, oranges, fennel, and the other ingredients in a salad bowl, stir and serve for breakfast.

Nutrition: Calories 97 Fat: 9.1g Carbs: 3.7g Protein: 1.9g

2.38 Raspberries and Yogurt Smoothie

Prep Time: 5 mins

Cook Time: 0 mins

Servings: 2

Ingredients:

- 2 cups raspberries
- ½ cup Greek yogurt
- ½ cup almond milk
- ½ tsp vanilla extract

Directions:

1. Blend the raspberries with the milk, vanilla, and yogurt in a blender until smooth, split into two glasses and serve for breakfast.

Nutrition: Calories 245 Fat: 9.5g Carbs: 5.6g Protein: 1.6g

2.39 Homemade Muesli

Prep Time: 15 mins

Cook Time: 20 mins

Servings: 8

Ingredients:

- 3 ½ cups rolled oats
- ½ cup wheat bran
- ½ tsp kosher salt
- ½ tsp ground cinnamon
- ½ cup sliced almonds
- ¼ cup raw pecans, coarsely chopped
- ¼ cup raw pepitas (shelled pumpkin seeds)
- ½ cup unsweetened coconut flakes
- ¼ cup dried apricots, coarsely chopped
- ¼ cup dried cherries

Directions:

1. Combine the oats, wheat bran, salt, and cinnamon in a medium mixing basin. Stir everything together well. Place the mixture on a baking sheet and set it aside.
2. After that, throw the almonds, pecans, and pepitas onto a separate baking sheet. Preheat your oven to around 350°F and place both trays inside. Preheat oven to 350°F and bake for 10-12 mins. Remove the pan from the oven and set it aside.
3. Allow the nuts to cool before removing the one with the oats and returning it to the oven for another 5 mins. Remove from the oven and set aside to cool.
4. Blend the contents of both trays in a large mixing basin and whisk well to combine. Stir in the apricots and cherries well. Place in an airtight container until ready to use.

Nutrition: Calories 250 Fat: 10g Carbs: 36g Protein: 7g

2.40 Tangerine and Pomegranate Breakfast Fruit Salad

Prep Time: 15 mins

Cook Time: 20 mins

Servings: 5

Ingredients:

- For the grains:
- 1 cup pearl or hulled barley
- 3 cups of water
- 3 tbsp. Olive oil, divided
- ½ tsp kosher salt
- For the fruit:
- ½ large pineapple, peeled and cut into 1 ½" chunks
- 6 tangerines
- 1 ¼ cups pomegranate seeds
- 1 small bunch of fresh mint
- For the dressing:
- 1/3 cup honey
- Juice and finely grated zest of 1 lemon

- Juice and finely grated zest of 2 limes
- ½ tsp kosher salt
- ¼ cup olive oil
- ¼ cup toasted hazelnut oil (olive oil is fine too)

Directions:

1. Rinse the grain well in a sieve. Place the grain on two baking pans that have been lined with parchment paper. Allow drying after spreading evenly.
2. After that, put the water in a pot and cook it over medium heat. 2 tbsp. Butter in a pan over medium heat. After that, add the barley to the oil. 2 mins of toasting
3. Bring the water, salt, and sugar to a boil. Reduce to low heat and cook for 40 mins, or until the liquid has almost been absorbed. Turn off the heat and set aside for 10 mins to steam cook the other ingredients.
4. Meanwhile, combine the honey, juices, zest, and salt in a medium mixing dish and toss well. Stir in the olive oil and then the nut oil. Place in the refrigerator until required.
5. Remove the cover of the barley and lay it on another baking sheet lined with parchment paper to cool. Drizzle with oil and set aside to cool fully before storing in the refrigerator.
6. Divide the grains, pineapple, orange, pomegranate, and mint amongst the bowls when ready to serve. Drizzle with the dressing before serving.

Nutrition: Calories 400 Fat: 23g Carbs: 50g Protein: 3g

CHAPTER 3:

Juice & Smoothies

3.1 Hot Tropical Smoothie

Prep Time: 5 mins.
Cook Time: 0 mins.
Servings: 4
Ingredients:

- 1 cup frozen mango chunks
- 1 cup frozen pineapple chunks
- 1 small tangerine, peeled and pitted
- 2 cups spinach leaves
- 1 cup coconut water
- ¼ tsp cayenne pepper, optional

Directions:

1. Add all ingredients and blitz until smooth and thoroughly combined in a food processor.
2. Serve right away or set aside for an hour to cool before serving.

Nutrition: Calories: 283 Fat: 1.9g Carbs: 67.9g Protein: 6.4g

3.2 Cranberry and Banana Smoothie

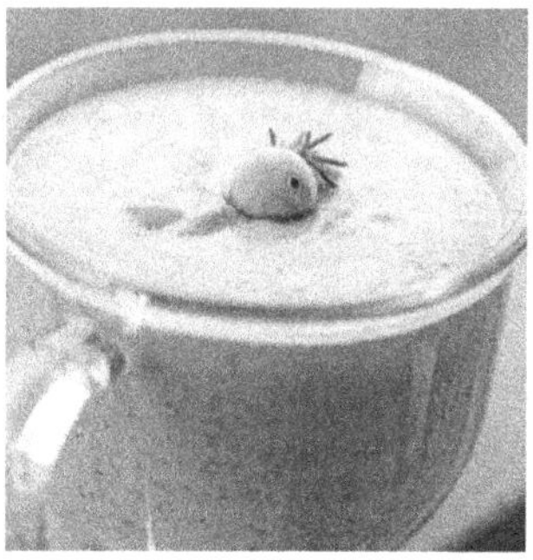

Prep Time: 5 mins.
Cook Time: 0 mins.
Servings: 4
Ingredients:

- 1 cup frozen cranberries
- 1 large banana, peeled
- 4 Medjool dates, pitted and chopped
- 1(½) cup unsweetened almond milk

Directions:

1. In a food processor, combine all ingredients and process until the mixture is glossy and thoroughly combined.
2. Serve right away or set aside for an hour to cool before serving.

Nutrition: Calories: 616 Fat: 8.0g Carbs: 132.8g Protein: 15.7g

3.3 Super Smoothie

Prep Time: 5 mins.
Cook Time: 0 mins.
Servings: 4
Ingredients:

- 1 banana, peeled
- 1 cup chopped mango
- 1 cup raspberries
- ¼ cup rolled oats
- 1 carrot, peeled
- 1 cup chopped fresh kale
- 2 tbsp chopped fresh parsley
- 1 tbsp flaxseeds
- 1 tbsp grated fresh ginger
- ½ cup unsweetened soy milk
- 1 cup water

Directions:

1. Combine all ingredients and blitz until glossy and smooth in a food processor.
2. Serve right away or set aside for an hour to cool before serving.

Nutrition: Calories: 550 Fat: 39.0g Carbs: 31.0g Protein: 13.0g

3.4 Kiwi and Strawberry Smoothie

Prep Time: 5 mins.
Cook Time: 0 mins.
Servings: 3
Ingredients:

- 1 kiwi, peeled
- 5 medium strawberries
- ½ frozen banana

- 1 cup unsweetened almond milk
- 2 tbsp hemp seeds
- 1 to 2 tsp maple syrup
- ½ cup spinach leaves
- Handful broccoli sprouts

Directions:

1. Combine all ingredients and blitz until creamy and smooth in a food processor.
2. Serve right away or set aside for an hour to cool before serving.

Nutrition: Calories: 562 Fat: 28.6g Carbs: 63.6g Protein: 23.3g

3.5 Banana and Chai Chia Smoothie

Prep Time: 5 mins.

Cook Time: 0 mins.

Servings: 3

Ingredients:

- 1 banana - 1 cup alfalfa sprouts
- 1 tbsp chia seeds
- ½ cup unsweetened coconut milk
- 1 to 2 soft Medjool dates, pitted
- ¼ tsp ground cinnamon
- 1 tbsp grated fresh ginger
- 1 cup water
- Pinch ground cardamom

Directions:

1. In a blender, combine all the ingredients & blend unless smooth and creamy. If required, add more water or coconut milk. Serve right away.

Nutrition: Calories: 477 Fat: 41.0g Carbs: 31.0g Protein: 8.0g

3.6 Summer Smoothie

Prep Time: 5 Mins

Cook Time: 5 mins

Servings 1

Ingredients:

- 1/2 cup Greek yogurt
- 2 cups raspberries
- 1 nectarine - 1 cup ice

Directions:

1. Combine all ingredients in a blender and mix until smooth.
2. Pour the smoothie into a glass and serve immediately.

Nutrition: Calories: 140 Carbs: 7g Fat: 13g Protein: 1g

3.7 Green Smoothie

Prep Time: 5 Mins

Cook Time: 5 mins

Servings 1

Ingredients:

- 1 cup almond milk
- 1 tbsp honey
- 1 banana
- 2 cups spinach
- 1/4 cucumber

Directions:

1. Combine all ingredients in a blender and process until smooth.
2. In a glass, pour the smoothie and serve.

Nutrition: Calories: 238 Fat: 12g Protein: 1g Carbs: 35g

3.8 Tropical Smoothie

Prep Time: 5 Mins

Cook Time: 5 mins

Servings 1

Ingredients:

- 1 banana
- 1 pineapple
- 1 cup mango
- 1 cup almond milk

Directions

1. In a blender, combine all the ingredients and process until smooth.
2. Strain the smoothie into a glass and serve.

Nutrition: Calories: 191 Fat: 14g Protein: 5g Carbs: 13g

3.9 Berry Smoothie

Prep Time: 5 Mins

Cook Time: 5 mins

Servings 1

Ingredients:

- 1 banana
- 4 cups pineapple juice
- 1 cup ice
- 4 oz. blueberries
- 4 oz. blackberries
- 1 tbsp honey

Directions

1. In a blender, combine all the ingredients and process until smooth.
2. Strain the smoothie into a glass and serve.

Nutrition: Calories: 193 Fat: 14g Protein: 1g Carbs: 18g

3.10 Citrus Smoothie

Prep Time: 5 Mins

Cook Time: 5 mins

Servings 1

Ingredients:

- 1 cup carrot juice - 1 banana
- 1 cup pineapple juice
- 1 cup ice

Directions

1. In a blender, combine all the ingredients and process until smooth.
2. Strain the smoothie into a glass and serve.

Nutrition; Calories: 101 Fat: 0g Protein: 1g Carbs: 27g

3.11 Pomegranate Smoothie

Prep Time: 5 Mins

Cook Time: 5 mins

Servings 1

Ingredients:

- 1 cup pomegranate juice
- 1 cup yogurt - 1 cup berries
- 1 cup ice - 1 cinnamon

Directions

1. In a blender, combine all the ingredients and process until smooth.
2. Strain the smoothie into a glass and serve.

Nutrition Calories: 97 Fat: 0g Protein: 3g Carbs: 23g

3.12 Mango Smoothie

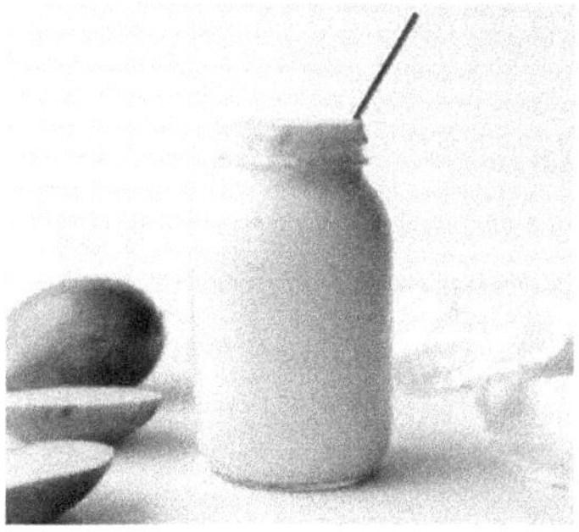

Prep Time: 5 Mins

Cook Time: 5 mins

Servings 1

Ingredients:

- 1 cup orange juice
- 1/4 cup vanilla yogurt
- 1 cup mango
- 1 carrot - 1 cup Ice

Directions

1. In a blender, combine all the ingredients and process until smooth.
2. Strain the smoothie into a glass and serve.

Nutrition: Calories: 367 Fat: 24.9g Protein: 26.6g Carbs: 13.7g

3.13 Green Citrus Smoothie

Prep Time: 10 Mins

Cook Time: 0 Mins

Servings: 2

Ingredients:

- 1 cup chopped watercress
- 1 large grapefruit, peeled
- 2 medium oranges, peeled
- 1 medium banana, peeled
- 1 cup water, divided

Directions:

1. In a blender, add the watercress, grapefruit, oranges, banana, and 1/2 cup water & blend unless smooth.
2. Blend in the remaining water until the desired texture is attained.

Nutrition: Calories: 162 Fat: 1g Protein 3g Carbs 41g

3.14 Cherry Pear Smoothie

Prep Time: 10 Mins

Cook Time: 0 Mins

Servings: 2

Ingredients:

- 1 cup chopped iceberg lettuce
- 2 medium pears, cored
- 1 medium banana, peeled
- 1/2 cup pitted cherries
- 1/2 tsp vanilla bean pulp
- 2 cups unsweetened vanilla almond milk, divided

Directions:

1. In a blender, add the vanilla pulp, banana, cherries, lettuce, pears, & almond milk, then blend unless smooth.
2. Blend in the leftover almond milk until the desired consistency is obtained.

Nutrition: Calories: 215 Fat: 3g Protein: 3g Carbs: 48g

3.15 Smoothie Apple Peach

Prep Time: 10 Mins

Cook Time: 0 Mins

Servings: 4

Ingredients:

- 2 tbsp rolled oats
- 1 cup chopped watercress

- 2 medium peaches, pitted
- 2 medium apples, cored and peeled
- 2 cups unsweetened vanilla almond milk, divided

Directions:

1. In a blender, add the oats, watercress, peaches, apples, and 1 cup almond milk & blend unless smooth.
2. Blend in the remaining almond milk until the desired texture is obtained.

Nutrition: Calories: 198 Fat: 4g Protein: 4g Carbs: 43g

3.16 Zucchini Apple Smoothie

Prep Time: 10 Mins

Cook Time: 0 Mins

Servings: 2

Ingredients:

- 1 cup spinach
- 1 medium zucchini, chopped
- 3 medium carrots, peeled and chopped
- 2 medium apples, cored and peeled
- 2 cups water, divided

Directions:

1. In a blender, add the spinach, zucchini, carrots, apples, and 1 cup water & blend unless smooth.
2. Blend in the remaining water until the desired texture is attained.

Nutrition: Calories: 163 Fat: 1g Protein: 4g Carbs: 40g

3.17 Farmers' Market Smoothie

Prep Time: 10 Mins

Cook Time: 0 Mins

Servings: 2

Ingredients:

- 1 cup chopped romaine lettuce
- 2 medium tomatoes
- 1 medium zucchini, chopped
- 2 medium stalks celery, chopped
- 1 medium cucumber, chopped
- 1/2 cup chopped green onions
- 2 cloves garlic, peeled
- 2 cups water, divided

Directions:

1. In a blender, mix garlic, romaine, tomatoes, cucumber, zucchini, celery, green onions, & water, then blend unless smooth.
2. If necessary, add the remaining 1 cup water while mixing until the desired viscosity is reached.

Nutrition: Calories: 85 Fat: 1g Protein: 5g Carbs: 17g

3.18 Smoothie Sweet Asparagus

Prep Time: 10 Mins

Cook Time: 0 Mins

Servings: 2

Ingredients:

- 1 cup chopped watercress
- 1 cup chopped asparagus
- 1 small lemon, peeled
- 1 large orange, peeled
- 1 cup water, divided

Directions:

1. In a blender, add the watercress, asparagus, lemon, orange, and 1/2 cup water & blend unless smooth.
2. Blend in the remaining water until the desired texture is attained.

Nutrition: Calories: 65 Fat: 0g Protein: 3g Carbs: 16g

3.19 Orange Broccoli Smoothie

Prep Time: 10 Mins

Cook Time: 0 Mins

Servings: 2

Ingredients:

- 1 cup chopped romaine lettuce
- 1 cup chopped broccoli
- 1 medium zucchini, chopped
- 2 medium carrots, peeled and chopped
- 2 cups water, divided

Directions:

1. In a blender, add the romaine, broccoli, zucchini, carrots, and 1 cup water & blend unless smooth.
2. Blend in the remaining water until the desired texture is attained.

Nutrition: Calories: 71 Fat: 1g Protein: 4g Carbs: 15g

3.20 Sweet Citrus Smoothie

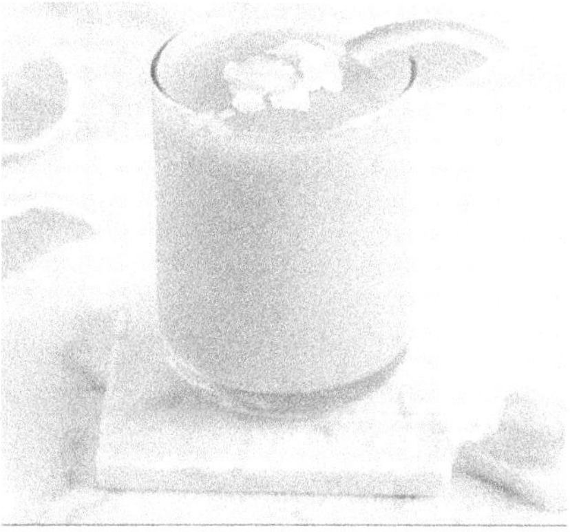

Prep Time: 10 Mins

Cook Time: 0 Mins

Servings: 2

Ingredients:

- 1 cup chopped watercress
- 1 large grapefruit, peeled
- 2 medium oranges, peeled
- 1 (1/2) piece ginger root, peeled
- 1/2 medium lemon, peeled
- 1 cup water, divided

Directions:

1. In your blender, add the oranges, ginger root, watercress, grapefruit, lemon, & water, then blend unless smooth.
2. Blend in the remaining water until the desired viscosity is attained.

Nutrition: Calories: 135 Fat: 0g Protein: 3g Carbs: 35g

3.21 The Smoothie Green Go-Getter

Prep Time: 10 Mins

Cook Time: 0 Mins

Servings: 1

Ingredients:

- 1 cup spinach
- 2 medium green apples, peeled and cored
- 1/2 medium banana, peeled
- 1 cup water, divided

Directions:

1. In a blender, add the spinach, apples, banana, and 1/2 cup water & blend unless smooth.
2. Continuc mixing while adding the remaining water until the desired texture is reached.

Nutrition: Calories: 241 Fat: 1g Protein: 2g Carbs: 63g

3.22 Clementine Smoothie

Prep Time: 5 Mins

Cook Time: 5 mins

Servings 1

Ingredients:

- 4 oz. clementine juice
- 2 oz. oats
- 2 oz. blueberries
- 2 pears
- 1 tbsp honey
- 1 tsp. mixed spice

Directions

1. Combine all ingredients in a blender and mix until smooth.
2. Pour the smoothie into a glass and serve immediately.

Nutrition: Calories: 86 Fat: 1g Protein: 5g Carbs: 17g

3.23 Avocado Smoothie

Prep Time: 5 Mins

Cook Time: 5 mins

Servings 1

Ingredients:

- 1 banana
- 2 tbsp cacao powder
- 1 tsp. coconut oil
- 1 avocado
- 1 tsp. vanilla extract
- 2 tbsp honey
- 1 cup ice

Directions

1. Combine all ingredients in a blender and mix until smooth.
2. Pour the smoothie into a glass and serve immediately.

Nutrition: Calories: 185 Fat: 7g Protein: 3g Carbs: 29g

3.24 Pear Smoothie

Prep Time: 5 Mins

Cook Time: 5 mins

Servings 1

Ingredients:

- 2 pears
- 1 banana
- 1 cup almond milk
- 1/2 cup vanilla yogurt
- 1 tsp. cinnamon

Directions

1. Combine all ingredients in a blender and mix until smooth.
2. Pour the smoothie into a glass and serve immediately.

Nutrition: Calories: 32 Carbs: 2g Fat: 0.1g Protein: 1g

3.25 Breakfast Smoothie

Prep Time: 5 Mins

Cook Time: 5 mins

Servings 1

Ingredients:

- 1 banana
- 1 tsp. coffee
- 1 tsp. cinnamon
- 1 tsp. honey
- 1 cup milk

Directions

1. Combine all ingredients in a blender and mix until smooth.
2. Pour the smoothie into a glass and serve immediately.

Nutrition: Calories: 140 Carbs: 7g Fat: 13g Protein: 1g

3.26 Banana Smoothie

Prep Time: 5 Mins

Cook Time: 5 mins

Servings 1

Ingredients:

- 2 tbsp cocoa powder
- 1 cup ice
- 1 banana
- 1 cup skimmed milk

Directions

1. Combine all ingredients in a blender and mix until smooth.
2. Pour the smoothie into a glass and serve immediately.

Nutrition: Calories: 193 Fat: 14g Protein: 1g Carbs: 18g

3.27 Green Juice Smoothie

Prep Time: 5 Mins

Cook Time: 5 mins

Servings 1

Ingredients:

- 2 apples
- 2 celery sticks
- 1 cucumber
- 1/2 cup kale leaves
- 1/4 lemon

Directions

1. Combine all ingredients in a blender and mix until smooth.
2. Pour the smoothie into a glass and serve immediately.

Nutrition: Calories: 86 Fat: 1g Protein: 5g Carbs: 17g

3.28 Spicy Smoothie

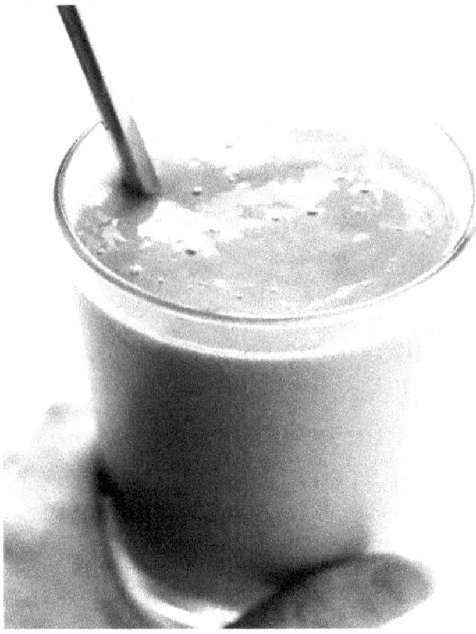

Prep Time: 5 Mins

Cook Time: 5 mins

Servings 1

Ingredients:

- 1 banana
- 2 oz. baby spinach
- 1 cup mango
- 1/4 tsp. jalapeno pepper
- 1 cup water

Directions

1. Combine all ingredients in a blender and mix until smooth.
2. Pour the smoothie into a glass and serve immediately.

Nutrition: Calories: 528 Fat: 39g Carbs: 25g Protein: 9g

3.29 Coconut Smoothie

Prep Time: 5 Mins

Cook Time: 5 mins

Servings 1

Ingredients:

- 1 mango
- 1 banana
- 1 cup coconut milk

- 1 cup pineapple chunks
- 2 tbsp coconut flakes

Directions

1. Combine all ingredients in a blender and mix until smooth.
2. Pour the smoothie into a glass and serve immediately.

Nutrition: Calories: 140 Carbs: 7g Fat: 13g Protein: 1g

3.30 Simple Smoothie Superfood

Prep Time: 5 Mins

Cook Time: 5 mins

Servings 2

Ingredients:

- 2 tsp. Chia seeds
- 1 tbsp. Matcha green tea powder
- 1 cup of fresh spinach for the baby
- 1 cup of frozen banana chopped
- 1/2 c. of chilled unpleasantly chopped almond milk
- 1 c. of fresh and fresh kale chopped
- 1/2 c. of frozen bananas chunks

Directions:

1. Pulse all ingredients smoothly in a high-speed blender.
2. Immediately serve with 2 large glasses of portion.

Nutrition: Calories: 65 Fat: 0g Protein: 3g Carbs: 16g

CHAPTER 4:

Soup & Salads

4.1 Brunoise Salad

Prep Time: 10 Mins
Cook Time: 0 Mins
Servings: 2

Ingredients:

- 1 tomato
- 1 zucchini
- ½ red bell pepper
- ½ yellow bell pepper
- ½ red onion
- 3 springs fresh parsley
- ½ lemon
- 2 tbsp. olive oil

Directions:

1. To make a brunoise, finely diced tomatoes, zucchini, peppers, and red onions. In a mixing dish, combine all the cubes. Chop the parsley and toss it in with the salad. Pour the olive oil over the salad and squeeze the lemon over it.
2. Add salt and pepper to taste.

Nutrition: Calories: 84 Carbs: 3g Fat: 4g Protein: 0g

4.2 Brussels Sprouts and Ricotta Salad

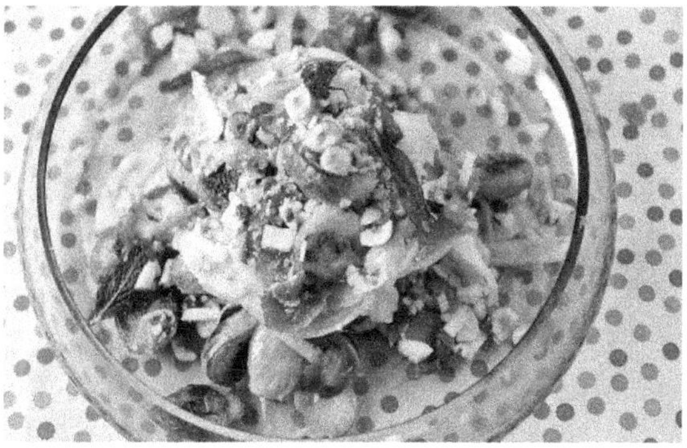

Prep Time: 15 Mins
Cook Time: 0 Mins
Servings: 2

Ingredients:

- 1 ½ cups Brussels sprouts, thinly sliced
- 1 green apple cut "à la julienne."
- ½ red onion
- 8 walnuts, chopped
- 1 tsp. extra-virgin olive oil
- 1 tbsp. lemon juice
- 1 tbsp. orange juice
- 4 oz. ricotta cheese

Directions:

1. Place the red onion in a cup and pour boiling water over it. Allow for 10 mins of resting time before draining and patting dry with kitchen paper. Slice the Brussels sprouts as thinly as possible, then cut the apple into julienne strips (sticks).
2. Combine Brussels sprouts, onion, and apple on a serving platter and season with oil, salt, pepper, lemon juice, and orange juice.
3. Top Brussels sprouts mixture with a tiny dollop of ricotta cheese and chopped walnuts.

Nutrition: Calories: 353 Fat: 4.8g Carbs: 28.1g Protein: 28.3g

4.3 Celery and Raisins Snack Salad

Prep Time: 10 Mins
Cook Time: 0 Mins
Servings: 4

Ingredients:

- ½ cup raisins
- 4 cups celery, sliced
- ¼ cup parsley, chopped
- ½ cup walnuts, chopped
- Juice of ½ lemon
- 2 tbsp. olive oil
- Salt and black pepper to taste

Directions:

1. Toss celery with raisins, walnuts, parsley, lemon juice, oil, and black pepper in a salad bowl.

2. Serve as a snack by dividing the mixture into small cups.

Nutrition: Calories: 120 Fat: 1g Carbs: 6g Protein: 5g

4.4 Dijon Celery Salad

Prep Time: 10 Mins

Cook Time: 0 Mins

Servings: 4

Ingredients:

- ½ cup lemon juice
- 1/3 cup Dijon mustard
- 2/3 cup olive oil
- Black pepper to taste
- 2 apples, cored, peeled, and cubed
- 1 bunch celery roughly chopped
- ¾ cup walnuts, chopped

Directions:

1. Mix celery and leaves with apple slices and walnuts in a salad dish.
2. Whisk together the black pepper, lemon juice, mustard, and olive oil, then add to your salad, stir, and serve in tiny cups.

Nutrition: Calories: 125 Fat: 2g Carbs: 7g Protein: 7g

4.5 Fresh Endive Salad

Prep Time: 10 Mins

Cook Time: 0 Mins

Servings: 1

Ingredients:

- ½ red endive
- 1 orange
- 1 tomato
- 1/2 cucumber
- 1/2 red onion

Directions:

1. Remove the endive leaves and cut off the firm stem. Cut the pulp into wedges after peeling the orange.
2. Tomatoes and cucumbers should be cut into tiny pieces. Thinly slice the red onion into half-rings.
3. Arrange the endive boats on a platter, then top with the orange wedges, tomato, cucumber, and red onion. Serve with a drizzle of olive oil and fresh lemon juice.

Nutrition: Calories: 112 Fat: 11g Carbs: 2g Protein: 0g

4.6 Green Creamy Soup

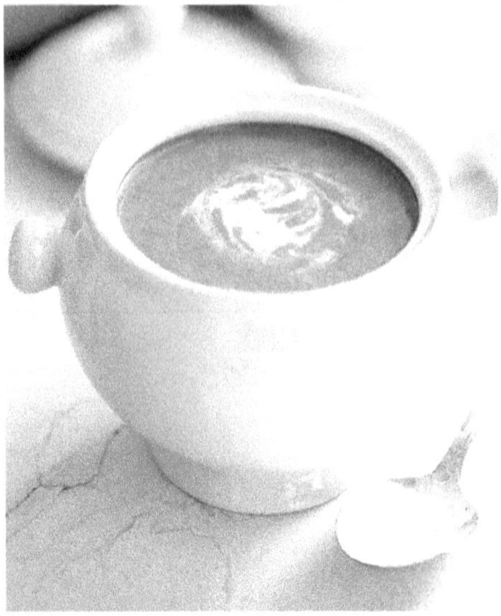

Prep Time: 10 mins

Cook Time: 30 mins

Servings: 2

Ingredients:

- 5 oz fresh pinto beans, thinly sliced
- 8 oz fresh Brussels sprouts, sliced
- 5 cups low-sodium, fat-free vegetable broth
- 1½ cups frozen peas, defrosted
- 4 tbsp olive oil
- 1 white onion, chopped
- 1 tbsp freshly squeezed lemon juice
- 4 cloves fresh garlic, minced
- 1 large leek, slice both white parts and sliced green parts thinly but keep them separate
- 1 tsp ground coriander
- 1 cup low-fat milk
- Salt and freshly ground pepper to taste
- Croutons for garnish

Directions:

1. Remove a big skillet from the oven and set it over low heat. Allow the olive oil to warm slightly before adding it.
2. Combine the onion and garlic in a bowl. Cook until the onions are aromatic and tender. Make sure they don't get brown when you're cooking them.
3. In a pan, combine the green pieces of the Brussels sprouts, leek, and pinto beans. Combine all ingredients, including the broth, in a large mixing bowl. Bring the broth to a boil over high heat. Reduce the heat to low and let it simmer for

approximately 12 mins until it begins to boil.

4. Combine the lemon juice, peas, and coriander in a mixing bowl. Allow for another 10 mins of simmering time or until the veggies are soft.
5. Remove the broth from the heat and set it aside to cool somewhat. Place the ingredients in a blender & blend unless smooth.
6. Remove the white sections of the leek and place them in a pot. Fill the pot halfway with the mixed mixture. Allow the soup to boil in the pot over medium-high heat. Reduce the heat to low and continue cooking the soup for another 5 minutes.
7. Remove another bowl and combine flour and milk in it. Whisk everything together until completely smooth.
8. If desired, season with salt and pepper to taste.

Nutrition: Calories: 163 Protein: 4 g Fat: 8 g Carbs: 15 g

4.7 Orzo and Lemon Chicken Soup

Prep Time: 10 mins

Cook Time: 40 mins

Servings: 2

Ingredients:

- 12 oz skinless, boneless chicken breasts
- 1 tbsp olive oil
- ½ cup chopped celery
- ½ cup chopped white onion
- 6 cups low-sodium, fat-free chicken broth
- ½ cup sliced carrot
- ½ cup orzo
- ¼ cup chopped fresh dill
- Salt and freshly ground pepper to taste
- Lemon halves

Directions:

1. Remove a big saucepan from the oven and set it over medium heat. Allow it to heat before adding the olive oil.
2. Toss in the celery and onion. Cook until the celery is tender, and the onions are aromatic.
3. Toss in the chicken, chicken stock, and carrots. If desired, season with salt & pepper.
4. Raise the heat to medium-high and allow the broth to come to your boil. Reduce the heat to low and let the soup to your simmer for 20 mins, or until the chicken is done.
5. Remove the chicken from the saucepan, place it in a basin, and set it aside to cool. Cover the saucepan and bring the contents to a low simmer. Shred-it into tiny pieces when the chicken is cold enough to handle.
6. Remove the lid from the saucepan and add the orzo. Increase the heat to medium-high and continue to cook the broth for approximately 8 mins. Make sure the lid is back on the pot during the boiling process.
7. Remove the saucepan from the heat and add the shredded chicken broth and dill.
8. Lemon juice should be squeezed into the soup. Serve right away.

Nutrition: Calories: 248 Protein: 25 g Fat: 4 g Carbs: 23 g

4.8 Chilled Avocado Soup

Prep Time: 50 mins

Cook Time: 0 mins

Servings: 2

Ingredients:

- 3 medium ripe seeded, peeled, avocados, halved
- 2 cloves fresh garlic, minced
- 2 cups low-sodium, fat-free chicken broth, divided
- ½ cucumber, chopped & peeled
- ½ cup white onion chopped
- ¼ cup carrot finely diced
- Thin avocado slices for garnish
- Paprika to sprinkle - Salt & pepper
- Hot red pepper sauce to taste

Directions:

1. Place 6 bowls in the freezer for half an hour to cool.
2. Meanwhile, combine the garlic, cucumber, avocados, onion, carrot, and 1 cup broth in a blender. Combine all the ingredients in a blender & blend unless smooth.
3. Pour in the rest of the broth. If desired, season to taste with salt, pepper, and spicy sauce. Re-blender all the ingredients until they are completely smooth.
4. Remove the cold dishes from the freezer and fill them with mixed ingredients.
5. Place the bowls in the refrigerator for another hour this time.
6. When ready to serve, sprinkle paprika and avocado slices over the soup.
7. Chill before serving.

Nutrition: Calories: 255 Protein: 4 g Fat: 22 g Carbs: 15 g

4.9 Broccoli and Potato Soup

Prep Time: 10 mins

Cook Time: 25 mins

Servings: 2

Ingredients:

- 2 cups escarole leaves, rinsed and drained
- 3 tbsp all-purpose flour
- 3 cups fresh broccoli florets
- 3 scallions, sliced
- 2 cups smoked Gouda cheese, shredded and more for garnish
- 2 cups low-sodium, fat-free chicken broth
- 1 cup almond milk
- 3 medium red-gold potatoes, chopped
- 2 cloves fresh garlic, minced
- Salt and freshly ground pepper to taste

Directions:

1. Remove a big saucepan from the oven and set it over medium-high heat. Combine the potatoes, garlic, and chicken stock in a large mixing bowl. Bring the mixture to a boil, then lower to a low heat setting. Allow the mixture to boil for a few mins, or until the potatoes soften.
2. Slightly mash the potatoes with a fork.
3. Combine the broccoli, milk, and scallions in a large mixing bowl. Continue to cook, occasionally stirring, until the broccoli is soft and crunchy.
4. Reduce the heat to low, then stir in the Gouda cheese. Stir until the sauce has thickened and the cheese has melted.
5. Season to taste with salt and pepper, if desired. Divide the soup into four equal servings and serve.
6. As toppers, add more cheese and escarole.

Nutrition: Calories: 350 Protein: 17 g Fat: 14 g Carbs: 42 g

4.10 Tortellini and Vegetable Soup

Prep Time: 10 mins

Cook Time: 30 mins

Servings: 2

Ingredients:

- 32 oz' low-sodium, fat-free chicken broth
- 3 cups fresh chicken-filled tortellini
- 1 large white onion, chopped
- 4 cloves fresh garlic, chopped
- 3 celery stalks, chopped
- 1 tsp minced chives
- 2 14.5-oz cans diced tomatoes, undrained
- 2 tbsp olive oil
- 1 tsp dried sweet basil
- 1 cup frozen corn
- 1 tsp dried thyme
- 1 cup chopped carrot
- 1 cup frozen cut pinto beans
- 1 cup diced raw potato

Directions:

1. Remove a big saucepan from the oven and set it over medium heat. Combine the garlic, onion, celery, and olive oil in a large mixing bowl. Sauté until the onion and garlic have softened and turned aromatic.
2. Potato, basil, carrot, beans, broth, thyme, corn, and chives are added to the saucepan. Bring the broth to a boil by increasing the heat to medium-high.
3. Reduce the heat and cover the pot after it begins to boil. Allow for a 15-min simmering period or until the veggies are soft.
4. Toss in the tortellini and tomatoes. Remove the lid and cook the soup for approximately 5 mins uncovered.
5. Serve immediately.

Nutrition: Calories: 213 Protein: 7 g Fat: 7 g Carbs: 26 g

4.11 Traditional Oyster Soup

Prep Time: 10 mins

Cook Time: 15 mins

Servings: 2

Ingredients:

- 2 pints (about 32 oz) freshly shucked oysters, undrained
- 4 tbsp olive oil
- 1 cup finely chopped celery
- 3 (12-oz) cans of low-fat evaporated milk
- 6 tbsp minced shallots
- 2 pinches of cayenne pepper (add more if you like more spice)
- Toasted bread squares
- Salt and freshly ground pepper to taste

Directions:

1. Let's begin with the oysters. In a small basin, drain the liquid from them. We're going to utilize the liquid, so set it aside. Oysters should be placed individually.
2. To eliminate any solids, strain the liquid using a filter.
3. Remove a big saucepan from the oven and set it over medium heat. Pour in some olive oil. Combine the oysters, celery, and shallots in a mixing bowl.

4. Allow the items to boil for 5 mins or until the oysters' edges curl.
5. Heat the oyster liquor and milk separately in a different pot (or pan). Pour the mixture over the oysters after it has reached the desired temperature. Combine all the ingredients in a mixing bowl.
6. Season with salt and pepper, as well as cayenne pepper, to taste.
7. Warm soup may be served with toasted bread pieces on top or the side.

Nutrition: Calories: 311 Protein: 23 g Fat: 11 g Carbs: 22 g

4.12 Eggplant Soup

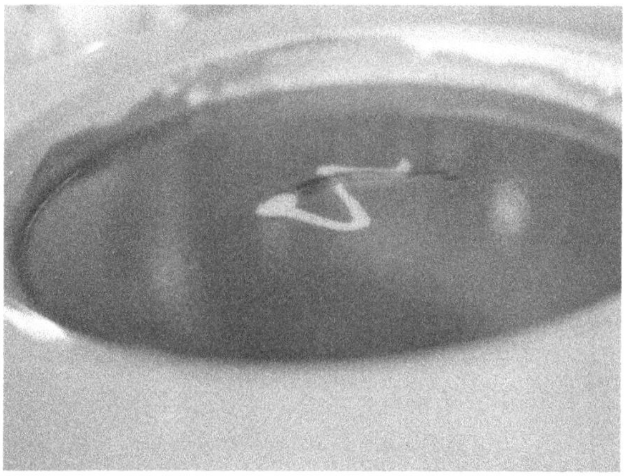

Prep Time: 10 mins

Cook Time: 30 mins

Servings: 2

Ingredients:

- 3 tbsp olive oil
- 1 (14-oz) can low-sodium tomato
- ½ cup chopped white onion
- 2 tbsp Italian breadcrumbs
- 2 cloves fresh garlic, minced
- 2 cups low sodium, fat-free chicken broth
- ½ cup shredded reduced-fat mozzarella cheese
- 1 small eggplant, halved and sliced thinly (about 2 cups)

Directions:

1. Preheat the oven to 500 degrees Fahrenheit. A broiling temperature is your goal. Broiling temperatures range from 500°F to 550°F in an oven.
2. If you wish to raise the temperature, do so when putting the dish in the oven.
3. Remove a nonstick pan from the oven and set it over medium heat. Allow the olive oil to heat up in the pan. Cook, stirring periodically, for approximately 5 mins after adding the eggplant.
4. Continue to sauté until the eggplant becomes a golden-brown hue, then add the garlic and onion.
5. Pour in the broth and the sauce. Allow the mixture to boil after increasing the heat to medium-high.
6. Reduce the heat to a gentle simmer after it begins to boil. Cook until the soup thickens, about 10 mins.
7. Remove a baking pan from the oven and line it with tin foil. Place two oven-safe crock bowls on the baking sheet. Pour the soup into the dishes, dividing it into equal pieces.
8. Breadcrumbs and mozzarella cheese are sprinkled on top.
9. Allow 2 to 3 mins for the dish to broil or until the cheese has melted and become brown.
10. Serve immediately.

Nutrition: Calories: 274 Protein: 9 g Fat: 17 g Carbs: 23 g

4.13 Cheesy Keto Zucchini Soup

Prep Time: 15 mins

Cook Time: 20 mins

Servings: 2

Ingredients:

- ½ medium onion, peeled and chopped
- 1 cup bone broth
- 1 tbsp coconut oil
- 1½ zucchinis, cut into chunks
- ½ tbsp nutritional yeast
- Dash of black pepper
- ½ tbsp parsley, chopped, for garnish
- ½ tbsp coconut cream, for garnish

Directions:

1. Melt the coconut oil and add the onions in a large pan over medium heat. Sauté for 3 mins before adding the zucchinis and bone broth.
2. Reduce the heat to low and cover the pan for approximately 15 mins. Transfer to an immersion blender with the nutritional yeast.
3. Season with black pepper & blend unless smooth. To serve, top with coconut cream and parsley.

Nutrition: Calories: 154 Carbs: 8.9g Fat: 8.1g Protein: 13.4g

4.14 Spring Soup with Poached Egg

Prep Time: 15 mins

Cook Time: 10 mins

Servings: 2

Ingredients:

- 32 oz vegetable broth
- 2 eggs
- 1 head romaine lettuce, chopped
- Salt, to taste

Directions:

1. Reduce the heat after bringing the vegetable broth to a boil. Remove the eggs from the broth after 5 mins and divide them between two dishes.
2. Cook for 4 mins after adding the romaine lettuce to the broth. Place in a dish and serve immediately.

Nutrition: Calories: 158 Carbs: 6.9g Fat: 7.3g Protein: 15.4g

4.15 Mint Avocado Chilled Soup

Prep Time: 15 mins

Cook Time: 0 mins

Servings: 2

Ingredients:

- 2 romaine lettuce leaves
- 1 Tbsp lime juice
- 1 medium ripe avocado
- 1 cup coconut milk, chilled
- 20 fresh mint leaves
- Salt to taste

Directions:

1. In a blender, combine all the ingredients and mix until smooth. Serve cooled after chilling for around 10 mins.

Nutrition: Calories: 432 Carbs: 16.1g Fat: 42.2g Protein: 5.2g

4.16 Easy Butternut Squash Soup

Prep Time: 15 mins

Cook Time: 1 hour & 35 mins

Servings: 4

Ingredients:

- 1 small onion, chopped
- 4 cups chicken broth
- 1 butternut squash
- 3 tbsp coconut oil
- Salt, to taste
- Nutmeg and pepper, to taste

Directions:

1. Combine the oil and onions in a large saucepan, then add the onions. Add chicken broth and butternut squash after 3 mins of sautéing.
2. Cook for 1 hour over medium heat before transferring to an immersion blender. Season with salt, pepper, and nutmeg after pulsing until smooth.
3. Cook for another 30 mins in the same pot. Remove the dish from the oven and serve immediately.

Nutrition: Calories: 149 Carbs: 6.6g Fat: 11.6g Protein: 5.4g

4.17 Cauliflower, Leek & Bacon Soup

Prep Time: 15 mins

Cook Time: 1 hour & 35 mins

Servings: 4

Ingredients:

- 4 cups chicken broth
- ½ cauliflower head, chopped
- 1 leek, chopped
- Salt and black pepper, to taste
- 5 bacon strips

Directions:

1. Cook for 1 hour on medium heat with the cauliflower, leek, and chicken broth in the pot. Pulse the mixture in an immersion blender until smooth.
2. Return the soup to the pot and cook the bacon strips for 1 min in the microwave. Place the bacon in the soup, cut it into tiny pieces.
3. Cook on low heat for around 30 mins. Serve with a pinch of salt and pepper.

Nutrition: Calories: 185 Carbs: 5.8g Fat: 12.7g Protein: 10.8g

4.18 Swiss Chard Egg Drop Soup

Prep Time: 15 mins

Cook Time: 10 mins

Servings: 4

Ingredients:

- 3 cups bone broth
- 2 eggs, whisked
- 1 tsp ground oregano
- 3 tbsp butter

- 2 cups Swiss chard, chopped
- 2 tbsp coconut aminos
- 1 tsp ginger, grated
- Salt and black pepper, to taste

Directions:

1. In a saucepan, heat the bone broth and carefully whisk in the beaten eggs. Combine the Swiss chard, butter, coconut aminos, ginger, oregano, salt, and black pepper in a large mixing bowl. Cook for 10 mins and serve immediately.

Nutrition: Calories: 185 Carbs: 2.9g Fat: 11g Protein: 18.3g

4.19 Mushroom Spinach Soup

Prep Time: 15 mins

Cook Time: 10 mins

Servings: 4

Ingredients:

- 1 cup spinach, cleaned and chopped
- 100g mushrooms, chopped
- 1onion
- 6 garlic cloves
- ½ tsp red chili powder
- Salt and black pepper, to taste
- 1 tsp almond flour
- 2 cups chicken broth
- 3 tbsp butter
- ¼ cup fresh cream for garnish
- **Direction**3 tbsp buttermilk

s:

1. In a pan, melt the butter and add the onions and garlic. After 3 mins of cooking, add the spinach, salt, and red chili powder.
2. After around 4 mins, add the mushrooms and continue to cook for another 4 mins. To produce a puree, transfer to a blender and mix until smooth. Return to the pan and add buttermilk and almond flour to get a creamy texture.
3. Stir everything up well and cook for around 2 mins. Serve immediately with a dollop of fresh cream on top.

Nutrition: Calories: 160 Carbs: 7g Fat: 13.3g Protein: 4.7g

4.20 Delicate Squash Soup

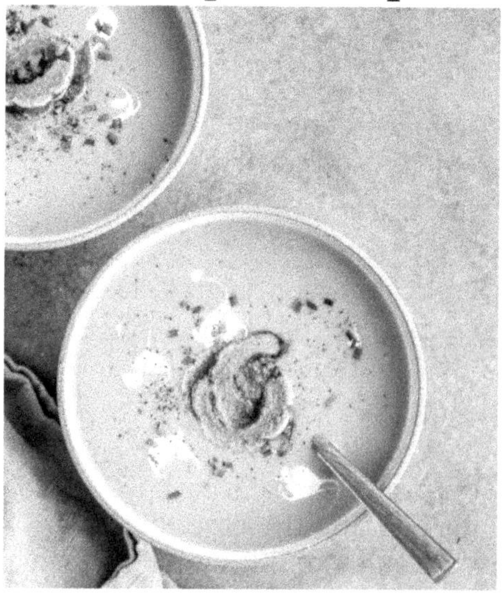

Prep Time: 15 mins

Cook Time: 27 mins

Servings: 5

Ingredients:

- 1½ cups beef bone broth
- 1small onion, peeled and grated.
- ½ tsp sea salt
- ¼ tsp poultry seasoning
- 2small Delicata Squash, chopped
- 2 garlic cloves, minced
- 2tbsp olive oil
- ¼ tsp black pepper
- 1 small lemon, juiced
- 5 tbsp sour cream

Directions:

1. In a medium saucepan, bring the Delicata Squash and water to a boil. Reduce the heat to low and continue to cook for another 20 mins. Drain the water and put it aside.
2. Combine the olive oil, onions, garlic, and poultry spice in a small saucepan. Cook for another 2 mins before adding the broth. Remove from heat after 5 mins of simmering.
3. Transfer the mixture to a blender after whisking in the lemon juice. Pulse till smooth, then serve with sour cream on top.

Nutrition: Calories: 109 Carbs: 4.9g Fat: 8.5g Protein: 3g

4.21 Broccoli Soup

Prep Time: 15 mins

Cook Time: 37 mins

Servings: 6

Ingredients:

- 3 tbsp ghee
- 5 garlic cloves
- 1 tsp sage
- ¼ tsp ginger
- 2 cups broccoli
- 1 small onion
- 1 tsp oregano
- ½ tsp parsley
- Salt and black pepper, to taste
- 6 cups vegetable broth
- 4 tbsp butter

Directions:

1. Cook for 3 mins in a saucepan with ghee, onions, spices, and garlic. Cook for 4 mins after adding the broccoli. Cover and cook for around 30 mins with the veggie broth.
2. Blend in a blender until completely smooth. Add the butter to give it a creamy, delightful texture and taste.

Nutrition: Calories: 183 Carbs: 5.2g Fat: 15.6g Protein: 6.1g

4.22 Keto French Onion Soup

Prep Time: 15 mins

Cook Time: 335 mins

Servings: 6

Ingredients:

- 5 tbsp butter
- 500 g brown onion medium
- 4 drops liquid stevia
- 4 tbsp olive oil
- 3 cups beef stock

Directions:

1. In a large saucepan over medium-low heat, melt the butter and olive oil, then add the onions and salt. Cook for 5 mins before adding the stevia.
2. Cook for a further 5 mins before adding the beef stock. Reduce to low heat and cook for approximately 25 mins. Pour into soup cups and serve immediately.

Nutrition: Calories: 198 Carbs: 6g Fat: 20.6g Protein: 2.9g

4.23 Cauliflower and Thyme Soup

Prep Time: 15 mins

Cook Time: 13 mins

Servings: 6

Ingredients:

- 2 tsp thyme powder
- 1 head cauliflower
- 3 cups vegetable stock
- ½ tsp matcha green tea powder
- 3 tbsp olive oil
- Salt and black pepper, to taste
- 5 garlic cloves, chopped

Directions:

1. Bring the vegetable stock, thyme, and matcha powder to a boil in a large saucepan over medium-high heat. Cook for approximately 10 mins after adding the cauliflower.
2. Meanwhile, heat the olive oil and garlic in a small saucepan for approximately 1 min. Cook for 2 mins after adding the garlic, salt, and black pepper.
3. Blend with an immersion blender until completely smooth. Remove the dish from the oven and serve right away.

Nutrition: Calories: 79 Carbs: 3.8g Fat: 7.1g Protein: 1.3g

4.24 Homemade Thai Soup

Prep Time: 15 mins

Cook Time: 8 hours

Servings: 12

Ingredients:

- 1 lemongrass stalk, cut into large chunks
- 5 thick slices of fresh ginger
- 1 whole chicken
- 20 fresh basil leaves
- 1 lime, juiced
- 1 tbsp salt

Directions:

1. A slow cooker combines the chicken, 20 basil leaves, lemongrass, ginger, salt, and water. Cook on low for 8 hours and then transfer to a bowl. To serve, add fresh lime juice and basil leaves.

Nutrition: Calories: 182 Carbs: 8.9g Fat: 9.3g Protein: 14.4g

4.25 Chicken Kale Soup

Prep Time: 15 mins

Cook Time: 6 hours & 15 mins

Servings: 6

Ingredients:

- 2 pounds' chicken breast, skinless
- 1/3cup onion
- 1 tbsp olive oil
- 14 oz' chicken bone broth
- ½ cup olive oil
- 4 cups chicken stock
- ¼ cup lemon juice

- 5 oz' baby kale leaves - Salt, to taste

Directions:

1. Season the chicken with black pepper and salt. Heat the olive oil over medium heat in a large pan and add the seasoned chicken.
2. Reduce the heat to low and cook for 15 mins. Place the chicken in the crock cooker after shredding it. Combine the chicken broth, onions, and puree in a blender until smooth.
3. Pour the remaining ingredients into the crockpot and stir to combine. Cook on low for 6 hours, stirring once throughout that time.

Nutrition: Calories: 266 Carbs: 33g Fat: 5.6g Protein: 22g

4.26 Chicken Veggie Soup

Prep Time: 15 mins

Cook Time: 1 hour & 30 mins

Servings: 6

Ingredients:

- 5 chicken thighs
- 12 cups water
- 1 tbsp adobo seasoning
- 4 celery ribs
- 1 yellow onion
- 1½ tsp whole black peppercorns
- 6 sprigs of fresh parsley
- 2 tsp coarse sea salt
- 2 carrots - 6 mushrooms, sliced
- 2 garlic cloves
- 1 bay leaf
- 3 sprigs fresh thyme

Directions:

1. Combine the water, chicken thighs, carrots, celery ribs, onion, garlic cloves, and herbs in a large saucepan. Bring to a boil, then lower to low heat.
2. Simmer for 30 mins with the lid on the pot. Remove the bones from the chicken and shred them. Return the bones to the stew and cook for another 20 mins.
3. Remove the pieces from the soup and strain the liquid back into the saucepan. Bring to a boil, then reduce to low heat for approximately 30 mins.
4. Simmer for around 10 mins with the mushrooms in the broth. Serve immediately after removing the dish from the oven.

Nutrition: Calories: 250 Carbs: 6.4g Fat: 8.9g Protein: 35.1g

4.27 Chicken Mulligatawny Soup

Prep Time: 15 mins

Cook Time: 30 mins

Servings: 10

Ingredients:

- 1½ tbsp curry powder
- 3 cups celery root, diced
- 2 tbsp Swerve
- 10 cups chicken broth
- 5 cups chicken, chopped and cooked
- ¼ cup apple cider
- ½ cup sour cream
- ¼ cup fresh parsley, chopped
- 2 tbsp butter
- Salt and black pepper, to taste

Directions:

1. Combine the broth, butter, chicken, curry powder, celery root, and apple cider in a large soup pot. Bring to a boil, then reduce to low heat for approximately 30 mins.
2. Swerve, sour cream, fresh parsley, salt, and black pepper are mixed. Remove the dish from the oven and serve immediately.

Nutrition: Calories: 215 Carbs: 7.1g Fat: 8.5g Protein: 26.4g

4.28 Buffalo Ranch Soup

Prep Time: 15 mins

Cook Time: 30 mins

Servings: 4

Ingredients:

- 2 tbsp parsley - 2 celery stalks, chopped
- 6 tbsp butter
- 1 cup heavy whipping cream
- 4 cups chicken, cooked and shredded
- 4 tbsp ranch dressing
- ¼ cup yellow onions, chopped
- 8 oz cream cheese
- 8 cups chicken broth
- 7 hearty bacon slices, crumbled

Directions:

1. In a skillet, melt the butter and add the chicken. Cook for 5 mins before adding 112 cups water. Cook for approximately 10 mins with the lid on.
2. Cook for around 10 mins with the chicken and the rest of the ingredients, except the parsley, in a saucepan. Serve immediately with parsley on top.

Nutrition: Calories: 478 Carbs: 7.5g Fat: 23.6g Protein: 56.6g

4.29 Traditional Chicken Soup

Prep Time: 15 mins
Cook Time: 1 hour & 30 mins
Servings: 6

Ingredients:

- 3 pounds' chicken
- 4 quarts' water
- 4 stalks celery
- 1/3 large red onion
- 1 large carrot
- 3 garlic cloves
- 2 thyme sprigs
- 2 rosemary sprigs
- Salt and black pepper, to taste

Directions:

1. In a stockpot over medium-high heat, combine the water and chicken. Bring to a boil, then reduce to low heat for approximately 10 mins.
2. Simmer for 30 mins on medium-low heat with onion, garlic, celery, salt, and pepper. Simmer for another 30 mins on low with the herbs and carrots.
3. Remove the bones from the chicken and shred the chunks. Add the rosemary sprigs to the saucepan with the chicken pieces. Simmer for around 20 mins on low heat before serving.

Nutrition: Calories: 314 Carbs: 3.3g Fat: 7g Protein: 66.2g

4.30 Noodle Soup

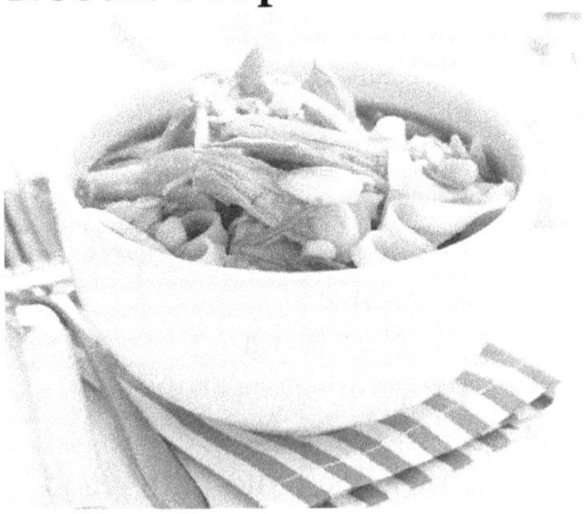

Prep Time: 15 mins
Cook Time: 20 mins
Servings: 6

Ingredients:

- 1 onion, minced
- 1 rib celery, sliced
- 3 cups chicken, shredded
- 3 eggs, lightly beaten
- 1 green onion for garnish
- 2 tbsp coconut oil
- 1 carrot, peeled and thinly sliced
- 2 tsp dried thyme
- 2½ quarts homemade bone broth
- ¼ cup fresh parsley, minced
- Salt and black pepper, to taste

Directions:

1. Heat the coconut oil over medium-high heat in a large saucepan and add the onions, carrots, and celery. Stir in the bone broth, thyme, and chicken after approximately 4 mins.
2. Cook for approximately 15 mins, then add the parsley. Slowly and steadily pour beaten eggs into the soup.
3. Remove the soup from the heat and set it aside for 2 mins. Season with salt and black pepper before serving.

Nutrition: Calories: 226 Carbs: 3.5g Fat: 8.9g Protein: 31.8g

4.31 Quinoa Pegan Salad Bowl

Prep Time: 15 Mins
Cook Time: 0 Mins
Servings: 4

Ingredients:

- Half cucumber
- 1 cup of cooked quinoa
- Half cup of canned black bean, rinsed
- 1/4 cup of diced onion
- 1 cup of baby spinach leaves
- Half cup of shredded purple Cabbage

Dressing

- 3 tsp of Lemon juice
- black pepper, to taste
- 1 tsp of miso gluten-free paste

Directions:

1. Toss all the veggies together in a bowl.
2. Whisk together the dressing ingredients in a separate dish.
3. Toss the salad with the dressing and serve.

Nutrition: Calories: 269 Fat: 7 g Carbs: 50 g Protein: 11 g

4.32 Slaw Salad

Prep Time: 15 Mins
Cook Time: 0 Mins
Servings: 4

Ingredients:

- 1 cup of arugula

- Half cup of shredded carrots
- Half can of roasted green peppers
- 1 cup of shredded green cabbage
- 1/4 cup of chopped green onion
- half sliced red onion
- half cup of shredded red cabbage
- 1/8 cup of chopped cilantro
- 2 tbsp of salad dressing
- 1 tbsp of chopped mint

Directions:

1. Combine all ingredients in a mixing bowl, stir, and serve.

Nutrition: Calories: 189 Fat: 2 g Carbs: 5 g Protein: 12 g

4.33 Bacon, Brussels Sprout & Spinach Salad

Prep Time: 15 Mins

Cook Time: 15 Mins

Servings: 4

Ingredients:

- 2 cups of Brussels sprouts, thinly sliced
- 3 tbsp of wine vinegar
- 1/4 tsp of sugar
- 3 tbsp of extra-virgin olive oil
- 1 1/2 tsp of caraway seed
- 8 slices of bacon
- Half-pound of chopped spinach

Directions:

1. Cook bacon until crispy in a pan, then crumble it on paper towels.
2. Cook for 1-2 mins with the Brussels sprouts in the pan with the seeds.
3. Except for the spinach, add the rest of the ingredients to the pan. 1 min of cooking
4. Cook for 1-2 mins after adding the spinach.
5. Add crispy bacon to the top just before serving. Serve.

Nutrition: Calories: 293 Fat: 19g Carbs: 12g Protein: 10g

4.34 Golden Beet & Potato Soup

Prep Time: 15 Mins

Cook Time: 45 Mins

Servings: 5-6

Ingredients:

- 2 tbsp of cooking oil
- 4 cups of water
- 1 lb. of peeled Russet potatoes, cubed
- 2 lbs. peeled golden beets & chopped
- 1 tsp of salt
- 2 sweet, chopped onions
- 1 tbsp of lemon juice
- 4 peeled garlic cloves
- black pepper, to taste

Directions:

1. Preheat the oven to 400 degrees Fahrenheit.
2. Toss the beets with half of the oil on a baking sheet and roast for 10 mins.
3. Spread onion, peeled garlic, and potatoes on a separate baking sheet, stir with the remaining oil, and roast for 30 mins.
4. Combine all roasted veggies, water, salt, and pepper in a pan.
5. Using a stick blender, puree the mixture.
6. Serve with lemon juice.

Nutrition: Calories: 265 Fat: 12 g Carbs: 13 g Protein: 14 g

4.35 Thai Mango Avocado Salad

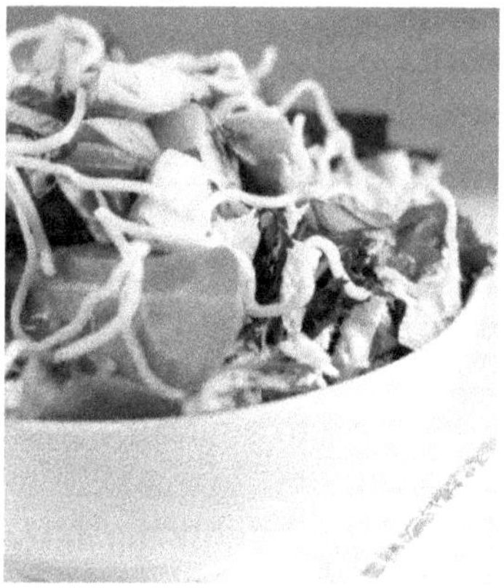

Prep Time: 15 Mins

Cook Time: 15 Mins

Servings: 5-6

Ingredients:

- 1 tbsp of Coconut Oil
- 1 cubed Avocado
- 1/4 cup of chopped Fresh Cilantro
- 1 cup of Mango - Sea Salt, to taste
- 1/4 cup of sliced Fresh Mint
- 1 peeled Sweet Potato & sliced into ¼" thick
- 2/3 cup of diced Cucumber

For Sauce:

- 2 tsp of paleo Fish Sauce
- 4 tsp of Lime Juice

Directions:

1. Preheat the grill to high.
2. Toss the potatoes in the oil, cook for 3 to 4 mins on one side, and then set aside to cool.

3. Transfer the potatoes to a basin and dice them.
4. Combine the remaining ingredients in a mixing bowl. Toss everything together and serve.

Nutrition: Calories 170 Fat: 8.2 g Carbs: 24.5 g Protein: 2.1 g

4.36 Warm Breakfast Salad

Prep Time: 10 Mins

Cook Time: 10 Mins

Servings: 4

Ingredients:

- 1/3 cup of diced shallot
- 1 tbsp of water
- 1 1/2 tbsp of olive oil
- 1/4 tsp of sea salt & pepper, each
- 1/3 cup of blueberries
- 1 1/3 cup of peeled butternut squash, chopped
- 12 oz. of Coleslaw mix
- 1 tbsp of balsamic vinegar
- 1 sliced avocado
- 1/4 tsp of minced garlic
- 4 eggs

Directions:

1. Microwave squash in a bowl with one tbsp of water for 2 to 2.5 mins, covered with plastic wrap.
2. Drain and thoroughly mash it.
3. 2 mins in a pan, sauté onion in heated oil. The remaining ingredients are combined except for the avocado, blueberries, eggs, and squash.
4. With one tbsp of water, cook for 1-2 mins.
5. Place it in a basin and top with blueberries.
6. Cook eggs to desired consistency, sunny side up.
7. Serve the slaw with eggs, avocado, and mashed squash.

Nutrition: Calories 235 Fat: 1.5 g Carbs: 18 g Fiber: 7g Sugar: 6.5 g Protein: 9.2 g Sodium: 213 mg

4.37 Grilled Chicken Taco Salad

Prep Time: 30 Mins

Cook Time: 20 Mins

Servings: 4

Ingredients:

- ¾ cup of salsa
- 1 cup of chopped cilantro, fresh
- 1 tsp of ground cumin
- 1 tbsp of lime juice
- 1 can of (15 oz.) black beans, rinsed
- 2 tbsp of chili powder
- 1 tsp of brown sugar
- 1 pound of chicken breast halved, skinless & boneless
- 1 tsp of ground coriander
- ¼ tsp of cayenne pepper
- 4 cups of shredded lettuce
- 1 tbsp of olive oil
- 4 corn tortillas of 7."

Directions:

1. Preheat the grill to medium-high and coat the grates with oil.
2. Toss the beans, half of the cilantro, lime juice, and salsa in a mixing bowl.
3. Combine the spices, oil, and sugar in a mixing dish and massage all over the chicken breasts.
4. Grill the chicken for 10-12 mins until it reaches an internal temperature of 165 degrees Fahrenheit.
5. For 3-5 mins, grill the tortillas.
6. Cut the chicken into strips and serve with the bean mixture and cilantro on the tortillas.

Nutrition: Calories: 470 Fat: 18.7 g Carbs: 44.4 g Protein: 35.2 g

4.38 Butternut Squash Soup

Prep Time: 10 Mins

Cook Time: 45 Mins

Servings: 6

Ingredients:

- 1 sweet, chopped onion
- 3 lbs. of peeled butternut squash, chopped
- 1 diced carrot
- 1 sprig of fresh thyme
- 1 diced celery rib
- 1 tbsp of olive oil
- 1 sprig of fresh rosemary
- 1/4 tsp of black pepper
- 3 cups of vegetable broth
- 1 peeled, chopped apple
- 3 minced garlic cloves
- 1/4 tsp of ground cinnamon
- 1 tsp of kosher salt

Directions:

1. For 3-5 mins, sauté the garlic, celery, carrots, and onion.

2. Add the other ingredients and simmer for 20-30 mins, or until the squash is soft; if it becomes dry, add additional broth.
3. Puree the soup with a stick blender and season to taste. Serve.

Nutrition: Calories: 159 Fat: 3 g Carbs: 36 g Protein: 3 g

4.39 Tuscan Black Cabbage Soup

Prep Time: 10 mins

Cook Time: 15 mins

Servings: 2

Ingredients:

- Pound Tuscan black cabbage
- Tbsp further virgin olive oil
- Large onion, thinly sliced
- Celery stalk, thinly sliced
- Carrot, diced
- Medium potato, bare-assed and diced
- 5 cups vegetable broth or water
- Salt - Freshly ground black pepper
- Slices wheaten bread
- Garlic cloves, peeled, and cut in half

Directions

1. Remove the stems from the cabbage and wash it. Remove the narrow strips and sauté the onion, celery, carrot, and potato for three mins in a large saucepan with vegetable oil.
2. Bring the cabbage and broth to a boil, then cover and simmer for one hour. After that, season it with salt and black pepper to taste.
3. Meanwhile, lay the pieces of bread on a baking sheet and toast in a preheated 375°F oven until golden.
4. Remove the slices from the cooking gadget and massage each one with garlic.
5. Place the bread pieces in separate soup bowls and top with the fresh soup.
6. Serve right away.

Nutrition: Calories: 456 Fat: 19g Carbs: 27g Protein: 8g

4.40 Potato Leek Soup

Prep Time: 10 mins

Cook Time: 20 mins

Servings: 5

Ingredients:

- 4 tbsp of olive oil
- 3 leeks
- 3 cups of onions, diced
- 1 lb. Of potatoes, diced
- 4 garlic cloves, chopped
- 1 tbsp of thyme
- 6 cups of veggie stock
- ½ tsp of pepper
- 1 tsp of salt
- ½ cup of plant-based sour cream
- 2 tbsp of chives for garnishing

Directions

1. Leeks should be cut in half lengthwise. Using a 14-inch round cutter, cut them into 14-inch rounds.
2. In a saucepan or oven, heat the oil over medium heat.
3. Sauté for 8 mins after adding the leeks.
4. Garlic should be included now. Continue to sauté for another 3 mins.
5. Combine the thyme, potatoes, and stock in a large mixing bowl. Boil. Reduce the heat to a low level and cook for 20 mins. Your potatoes should be cooked through.
6. Season with salt and pepper.
7. To make it silky and smooth, blend it in batches.
8. Put the soup back in the pot. Simmer on a low heat setting.
9. Toss with the sour cream. Garnish with chives.

Nutrition: Calories: 224 Carbs: 31g Fat: 13g Protein: 4g

CHAPTER 5:

Vegan Recipes

5.1 Zucchini with mixed herbs

- p dried mix herbs
- 1 garlic clove, minced
- 2 tbsp olive oil

Directions:

1. Preheat the oven to 450 degrees Fahrenheit/232 degrees Celsius. Toss all the ingredients together in a large mixing basin.
2. Transfer the zucchini mixture to the baking dish and bake for 10 mins in a preheated oven. Return to the oven and bake for another 5 mins. Serve and have fun.

Nutrition: Calories: 102 Fat: 8.7g Protein: 3.7g Carbs: 4.3g

5.2 Spaghetti Squash with Tomato Basil Cream

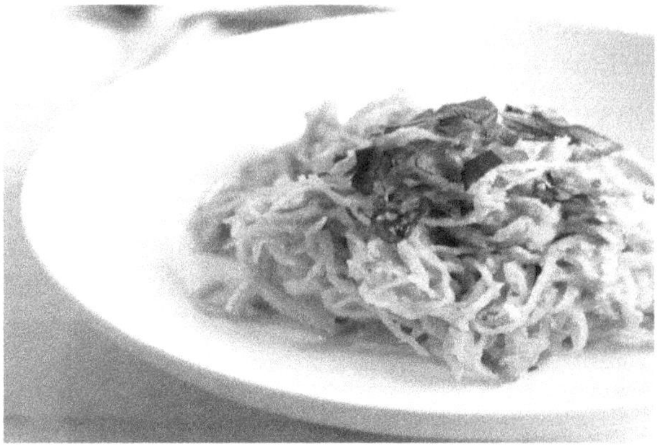

Prep Time: 10 mins

Cook Time: 15 mins

Servings: 4

Ingredients:

Spaghetti Squash:

- 1 spaghetti squash, medium
- Salt & pepper to taste
- 2 tsp of olive oil

Tomato sauce:

- 2 tbsp of water
- Half tsp of salt
- 1 can of (15 oz.) diced roasted tomatoes
- ¼ cup of chopped fresh basil
- Half cup of soaked cashews

Directions:

1. Preheat the oven to 375 degrees Fahrenheit.
2. Remove the seeds and membrane from the squash by cutting it in half.
3. Rub some olive oil into the squash and season with salt, garlic, and pepper.
4. Bake for 35 mins, face down, on a baking sheet.
5. Combine all ingredients in a blender and pulse until smooth to make the sauce.
6. To make spaghetti, shred the cooked spaghetti.
7. At a medium temperature, add oil to a pan. Toss in the spaghetti squash and sauce, and simmer for another 2-3 mins.
8. Serve.

Nutrition: Calories: 257 Fat: 12.9 g Carbs: 31 g Protein: 6 g

5.3 Vegan Shepherd's Pie

Prep Time: 15 Mins

Cook Time: 1 hour & 35 Mins

Servings: 6

Ingredients:

- Sea salt & black pepper, to taste
- 3 to 4 Tbsp of vegan butter
- 3 pounds of peeled Yukon potatoes

Filling:

- 1 chopped onion
- 1 1/2 cups of rinsed brown lentils
- 2 minced cloves garlic
- 1 tbsp of olive oil
- 4 cups of vegetable stock
- 2 tbsp of tomato paste
- 10 oz. of frozen mixed vegetables
- 2 pinches of sea salt & pepper, each
- 2 tsp of fresh thyme

Directions:

1. Boil water with a substantial quantity of salt in a saucepan.
2. Cook for 20 to 30 mins, covered, after adding the potatoes.
3. Drain and place in a mixing bowl. With vegan butter, salt, and pepper, mash the potatoes.
4. Preheat the oven to 425 degrees Fahrenheit. Spray a 2-quart baking dish with cooking oil.
5. Sauté garlic and onion in heated oil for 5 mins in a pan.
6. Cook for 1 min after adding tomato paste, salt, and pepper.
7. Stir with the remaining ingredients. Bring to a boil, then reduce to low heat and cook for 25 to 30 mins.
8. Cook for five mins after adding the frozen veggies.
9. Season to taste. Pour the mixture into the prepared dish, cover with mashed potatoes, spread with a fork, and season with salt and pepper.
10. Preheat oven to 350°F and bake for 10 to 15 mins. Serve.

Nutrition: Calories: 396 Fat: 1.6 g Carbs: 72 g Protein: 17.7 g

---

5.4 Creamy Carrot Soup

Prep Time: 10 mins

Cook Time: 45 mins

Servings: 6

Ingredients:

- 2 lb. Carrots, peeled and sliced
- 4 garlic cloves, chopped
- 2 leeks, sliced
- 2 tbsp olive oil
- 4 cups vegetable stock
- 1/2 tsp ground cumin
- 1/4 tsp ground coriander
- Pepper
- Salt

Directions:

1. In a medium saucepan, heat the olive oil. Cook for 15 mins with carrots, cumin, coriander, garlic, leek, pepper, and salt. Stir in the stock well. Bring the water to a boil.
2. Reduce the heat to low and cook for 30 mins. Using an immersion blender, puree the soup until it is completely smooth. Serve and have fun.

Nutrition: Calories: 125 Fat: 5.1g Protein: 1.9g Carbs: 20.2g

---

5.5 Zucchini Noodles with Avocado Sauce

Prep Time: 15 Mins

Cook Time: 0 Mins

Servings: 2

Ingredients:

- 1 1/4 cup of basil
- 1 avocado
- 1/3 cup of water
- 1 zucchini, spiralized into noodles
- 4 tbsp of pine nuts
- 12 cherry tomatoes, sliced
- 2 tbsp of lemon juice

Directions:

1. Combine all ingredients in a blender, except the zoodles and cherry tomatoes.
2. Combine the puree, zoodles, and tomatoes in a mixing basin. Serve after a thorough tossing.

Nutrition: Calories: 313 Fat: 26.8 g Carbs: 18.7 g Protein: 6.8 g

---

5.6 Avocado Tomato Salad

Prep Time: 10 mins

Cook Time: 0 mins

Servings: 4

Ingredients:

- 2 avocados, diced
- ½ onion, diced
- 1 tbsp olive oil
- ¼ cup fresh cilantro, chopped
- 1 fresh lime juice
- 4 cups cherry tomatoes, halved
- Pepper
- Salt

Directions:

1. Toss all the ingredients together in a mixing basin. Serve and have fun.

Nutrition: Calories: 276 Fat: 23.5g Protein: 3.7g Carbs: 17.9g

---

5.7 Vegan Vegetarian Curry

Prep Time: 15 Mins

Cook Time: 40 Mins

Servings: 6

Ingredients:

- 12 oz of cauliflower florets
- 10 oz of eggplants, cubed

- 1 diced bell pepper
- 1 tsp of coarse salt
- 10 oz of broccoli florets
- black pepper, to taste
- 6 tbsp of olive oil

Aromatics:

- 2 chopped shallots
- 2 tbsp of chopped garlic
- 1 tbsp of chopped ginger

Spices & Other:

- 1 to 1.5 tbsp of tamarind concentrate
- 14 oz of canned coconut milk
- 1 tsp of cumin, turmeric, and coriander powder
- 1 tbsp of almond butter

Directions:

1. Preheat the oven to 420 degrees Fahrenheit.
2. Vegetables should be spread out on a baking pan. Combine the salt, oil, and pepper in a mixing bowl.
3. On the middle rack, bake for 25 to 30 mins.
4. Add aromatics to a pan and cook for 2 mins in oil over medium heat.
5. Cook for 30 seconds after adding the spices.
6. Combine the remaining ingredients in a mixing bowl. Cook for a total of 2 to 3 mins.
7. Add the roasted veggies to the curry and toss to coat.
8. Serve.

Nutrition: Calories: 321 Fat: 12 g Carbs: 13.5 g Protein: 5.6 g

---

5.8 Creamy Polenta with Mushrooms

Prep Time: 15 mins

Cook Time: 30 mins

Servings: 2

Ingredients:

- ½ oz (14 g) dried porcini mushrooms (optional but recommended)
- 2 tbsp olive oil
- 1 pound (454 g) baby Bella (cremini) mushrooms, quartered
- 1 large shallot, minced
- 1 garlic clove, minced
- 1 tbsp flour
- 2 tsp tomato paste
- ½ cup red wine
- 1 cup mushroom stock (or reserved liquid from soaking the porcini mushrooms, if using)
- ½ tsp dried thyme
- 1 fresh rosemary sprig
- 1½ cups water
- ½ tsp salt
- 1/3 cup instant polenta

Directions:

1. If using dried porcini mushrooms, soak them for 15 mins in 1 cup boiling water to soften them.
2. Scoop them out of the water after they've softened, retaining the soaking liquid. Porcini mushrooms should be minced.
3. In a large sauté pan, heat the olive oil over medium-high heat. Sauté the mushrooms, shallot, and garlic for 10 minutes, or until the veggies are wilted and caramelized.
4. Cook for another 30 seconds after adding the flour and tomato paste. Combine the red wine, porcini soaking liquid, thyme, and rosemary in a large mixing bowl.
5. Bring to a boil, stirring continually, until the mixture thickens. Reduce the heat to low and let for a 10-min simmer. Meanwhile, in a saucepan, bring the water to a boil and season with salt.
6. Stir in the instant polenta immediately as it thickens. Taste and season with more salt if necessary. Warm the dish before serving.

Nutrition: Calories: 450 Fat: 16.0g Protein: 14.1g Carbs: 57.8g

---

5.9 Roasted Vegetables and Chickpeas

Prep Time: 15 mins

Cook Time: 30 mins

Servings: 2

Ingredients:

- 4 cups cauliflower florets (about ½ small head)
- 2 medium carrots, peeled, halved, and then sliced into quarters lengthwise
- 2 tbsp olive oil, divided
- ½ tsp garlic powder, divided
- ½ tsp salt, divided
- 2 tsp za'atar spice mix, divided
- 1 (15-oz / 425-g) can chickpeas, drained, rinsed, and patted dry
- 1 tsp harissa spice paste

Directions:

1. Preheat the oven to 400 degrees Fahrenheit (205 degrees Celsius). Using foil or parchment paper, line a sheet pan. In a large mixing basin, combine the cauliflower and carrots.
2. 1 tbsp olive oil, 14 tsp garlic powder, 14 tsp salt, and 1 tsp za'atar drizzled over the top.
3. Toss everything together well. Arrange the veggies in a single layer on one side of the sheet pan.
4. Season the chickpeas with the remaining 1 tbsp of oil, 14 tsp of garlic powder, 14 tsp of salt, and the remaining za'atar in the same dish. Toss everything together well.
5. On the opposite side of the sheet pan, spread the chickpeas.
6. Roast for 30 mins, or until the chickpeas become brown and the veggies are soft. Halfway through the cooking time, flip the veggies and toss the chickpeas to ensure equal cooking.
7. If you want your chickpeas crunchy, cook them for a few mins longer. If this is the case, remove the veggies and cook the chickpeas until they reach the required crispiness.
8. Taste and season with harissa, if preferred, before serving.

Nutrition: Calories: 468 Fat: 23.0g Protein: 18.1g Carbs: 54.1g

---

5.10 Mexican Roasted Cauliflower

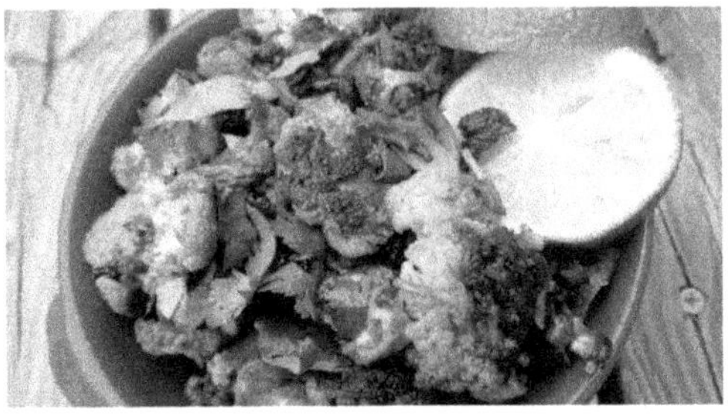

Prep Time: 15 Mins

Cook Time: 40 Mins

Servings: 4

Ingredients:

- 2 tbsp of avocado oil
- 1/4 cup of cilantro
- Half tsp of garlic powder
- 1 cauliflower, large head, broken into florets
- Half tsp of onion powder
- 1/4 tsp of cumin
- 1/4 cup of green onion sliced
- 1 tsp of chili powder
- 3/4 tsp of salt
- 1/4 tsp of pepper
- Half avocado, sliced
- 3 lime wedges

Directions:

1. Preheat the oven to 425 degrees Fahrenheit.
2. The onion, avocado, cilantro, and wedges, combine all ingredients in a mixing dish. Toss thoroughly and put on a baking sheet lined with parchment paper.
3. Bake for 20 minutes, then turn and roast for another 10 to 12 minutes.
4. On top of the onion, avocado, cilantro, and wedges serve.

Nutrition: Calories: 50 Fat: 4.0 g Carbs: 5.0 g Protein: 1.2 g

---

5.11 Roasted Leeks with red onion

Prep Time: 15 mins

Cook Time: 8 mins

Servings: 2

Ingredients:

- 3 tbsp olive oil
- 2 garlic cloves, crushed
- 2 leeks, chopped
- 2 red onions, chopped
- 9 oz (255 g) fresh spinach
- 1 tsp kosher salt

Directions:

1. Using the olive oil, coat the bottom of the big skillet. Stir in the garlic, leek, and onions for approximately 5 mins.
2. Add the spinach and mix well. Add the salt and continue to cook for another 3 mins, stirring regularly. Serve immediately on a platter.

Nutrition: Calories: 447 Fat: 31.2g Protein: 14.6g Carbs: 28.7g

---

5.12 Crispy Plantains with Garlic Sauce

Prep Time: 20 Mins

Cook Time: 25 Mins

Servings: 2-4

Ingredients:

Plantains:

- 1 to 2 tbsp of cooking oil
- Water, as needed
- 1 tbsp of salt

- 2 green plantains

Garlic Sauce:

- 1/3 cup of olive oil
- 1/4 tsp of salt, cumin seeds & red pepper flakes, each
- 1 scallion
- 2 cloves of garlic
- Half lime's juice

Directions:

1. Plantains should be peeled and sliced into one" thick slice.
2. Add plantain slices to a pan with enough water to cover them and salt.
3. Cover the pan, bring to a boil, then reduce to low heat and cook for 10 to 15 mins.
4. Combine all ingredients in a food processor and pulse until smooth to make the sauce.
5. Drain the plantains and softly mash them between paper towels, but not totally.
6. Cook plantain on one side for 3 to 5 mins in a skillet with oil. Season with salt to taste.
7. Garlic sauce is served on the side.

Nutrition: Calories: 78 Fat: 1.3 g Carbs: 3.1 g Protein: 2.4 g

5.13 Paleo Pizza Crust

Prep Time: 20 Mins

Cook Time: 25 Mins

Servings: 2-4

Ingredients:

- 1 tsp of avocado oil
- 2 tbsp of palm shortening
- 2 cups of mashed yuca
- Dried mixed herbs to taste
- 2 tbsp of coconut flour
- Half tsp of sea salt

Directions:

1. Preheat the oven to 375 degrees Fahrenheit.
2. Combine all ingredients (excluding flour) in a food processor and pulse until smooth.
3. Place it on parchment paper and sprinkle with coconut flour.
4. Divide the dough into two halves.
5. Roll each piece into a half-inch thick crust.
6. Bake for 15 to 20 mins, then turn and continue baking until golden brown.
7. Serve with chosen sauce and vegan cheese.

Nutrition: Calories: 86 Fat: 1 g Carbs: 4 g Protein: 2 g

5.14 Zucchini Crisp

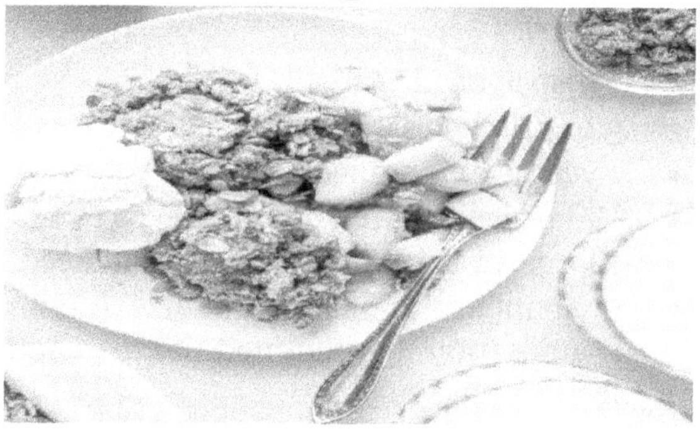

Prep Time: 15 mins

Cook Time: 20 mins

Servings: 2

Ingredients:

- 4 zucchinis, sliced into ½-inch rounds
- ½ cup unsweetened almond milk
- 1 tsp fresh lemon juice
- 1 tsp arrowroot powder
- ½ tsp salt, divided
- ½ cup whole wheat breadcrumbs
- ¼ cup nutritional yeast
- ¼ cup hemp seeds - ½ tsp garlic powder
- ¼ tsp crushed red pepper
- ¼ tsp black pepper

Directions:

1. Preheat the oven to 375 degrees Fahrenheit (190 degrees Celsius). Set aside two baking sheets lined with parchment paper.
2. Combine the zucchini, almond milk, lemon juice, arrowroot powder, and 14 tsp of salt in a medium mixing basin. Stir everything together well.
3. Combine the breadcrumbs, nutritional yeast, hemp seeds, garlic powder, crushed red pepper, and black pepper in a large mixing basin with a cover. Shake the zucchini slices in batches until they are uniformly covered.
4. Arrange the zucchini in a single layer on the prepared baking sheets. Bake for approximately 20 mins, or until the zucchini slices are golden brown, in a preheated oven.
5. Before serving, season with the remaining 14 tsp of salt.

Nutrition: Calories: 255 Fat: 11.3g Protein: 8.6g Carbs: 31.9g

5.15 Creamy Sweet Potatoes and Collards

Prep Time: 15 mins

Cook Time: 35 mins

Servings: 2

Ingredients:

- 1 tbsp avocado oil
- 3 garlic cloves, chopped
- 1 yellow onion, diced
- ½ tsp crushed red pepper flakes
- 1 large, sweet potato, peeled and diced
- 2 bunches collard greens (about 2 pounds/907 g), stemmed, leaves chopped into 1-inch squares
- 1 (14.5-oz / 411-g) can diced tomatoes with juice
- 1 (15-oz / 425-g) can red kidney beans or chickpeas, drained and rinsed
- 1½ cups water
- ½ cup unsweetened coconut milk
- Salt and black pepper, to taste

Directions:

1. Melt the avocado oil in a big, deep pan over medium heat. Cook for 3 mins after adding the garlic, onion, and red pepper flakes. Combine the sweet potato and collards in a mixing bowl.
2. Mix in the tomatoes, along with their juice, beans, water, and coconut milk. Just bring the mixture to a boil.
3. Reduce the heat to medium-low, cover, and cook for 30 mins or until the vegetables are softened. Season with salt and pepper to taste and serve.

Nutrition: Calories: 445 Fat: 9.6g Protein: 18.1g Carbs: 73.1g

5.16 Mediterranean Romaine Wedge Salad

Prep Time: 15 mins

Cook Time: 0 mins

Servings: 4

Ingredients:

- 1 English cucumber, chopped
- 1 cup quartered cherry tomatoes
- 1 cup chopped fennel
- ½ cup chopped roasted red peppers
- ¼ cup pitted, halved Kalamata olives
- 1 scallion, both white and green parts, chopped
- ½ cup Pesto Vinaigrette, divided
- 2 romaine lettuce heads, cut in half lengthwise
- 2 tbsp chopped fresh basil

Directions:

1. Combine the cucumber, tomatoes, fennel, roasted red peppers, olives, scallion, and 14 cup pesto vinaigrette in a large mixing basin.
2. On a big dish, place each romaine half. Distribute the veggie mixture evenly among the wedges. Over the romaine wedges, drizzle the remaining dressing. Serve with basil on top.

Nutrition: Calories: 336 Fat: 27g Carbs: 23g Protein: 11g

5.17 Roasted Brussels Sprouts and Halloumi Salad

Prep Time: 15 mins

Cook Time: 35 mins

Servings: 4

Ingredients:

- For the dressing:
- ¼ cup olive oil
- 1/3 cup freshly squeezed lemon juice
- 2 tbsp honey
- 1 tsp mustard
- Sea salt
- Freshly ground black pepper
- For the salad:
- 2 pounds Brussels sprouts, trimmed and halved
- 2 tbsp olive oil
- 1 tsp sea salt
- 1½ cups baby spinach
- ½ cup baby arugula
- 1 shallot, halved and thinly sliced
- 3 tbsp dried cranberries
- ½ cup blanched almonds, toasted
- ¼ cup shredded halloumi cheese

Directions:

1. Mix the olive oil, lemon juice, and mustard in a small bowl to make the dressing. Set aside after seasoning with salt and pepper.
2. To make the salad, combine all ingredients in a large mixing bowl.
3. Preheat the oven to 425 degrees Fahrenheit. In a large mixing dish, place the Brussels sprouts. Season with salt and drizzle with olive oil. Toss everything together.

4. On a large baking sheet, spread out the Brussels sprouts. Roast for 25 to 30 mins, until crispy on the exterior and soft on the inside, tossing once halfway through.
5. While the Brussels sprouts are roasting, combine the spinach, arugula, shallot, cranberries, and almonds in a large mixing bowl. Add the roasted Brussels sprouts to the bowl after they've finished cooking.
6. Toss the salad with the dressing to mix. Place the salad on a large serving plate to serve.

Nutrition: Calories: 475 Fat: 34g Carbs: 41g Protein: 14g

5.18 Roasted Vegetable Mélange

Prep Time: 15 mins

Cook Time: 25 mins

Servings: 4

Ingredients:

- ½ cauliflower head, cut into small florets
- ½ broccoli head, cut into small florets
- 2 zucchinis, cut into ½-inch pieces
- 2 cups halved mushrooms
- 2 red, orange, or yellow bell peppers, cut into 1-inch pieces
- 1 sweet potato, cut into 1-inch pieces
- 1 red onion, cut into wedges
- 3 tbsp olive oil - 2 tsp minced garlic
- 1 tsp chopped fresh thyme
- Sea salt - Freshly ground black pepper

Directions:

1. Preheat the oven to 400 degrees Fahrenheit. Set aside a baking sheet lined with parchment paper.
2. Toss the cauliflower, broccoli, zucchini, mushrooms, bell peppers, sweet potato, onion, olive oil, garlic, and thyme together in a large mixing bowl until thoroughly combined. Season the veggies liberally with salt and pepper and spread them out on the baking sheet. Roast for 20 to 25 mins, tossing periodically until the veggies are soft and faintly caramelized. Serve.

Nutrition: Calories: 183 Fat: 11g Carbs: 20g Protein: 5g

5.19 Couscous-Avocado Salad

Prep Time: 15 mins

Cook Time: 10 mins

Servings: 4

Ingredients:

- For the dressing:
- ¼ cup olive oil
- 2 tbsp red wine vinegar
- 1 tsp minced garlic
- 1 tsp chopped fresh oregano
- Pinch red pepper flakes
- Sea salt
- Freshly ground black pepper
- For the salad:
- 1 cup couscous
- 2 cups halved cherry tomatoes
- ½ English cucumber, chopped
- 1 cup chopped marinated artichoke hearts
- 1 avocado, pitted, peeled, and chopped
- 2 tbsp pine nuts

Directions:

1. Whisk together the olive oil, vinegar, garlic, oregano, and red pepper flakes in a small mixing dish to make the dressing. Set aside after seasoning with salt and pepper.
2. To make the salad, combine all ingredients in a large mixing bowl.
3. Bring 112 cups of water to a boil in a kettle. Remove the couscous from the heat after stirring it into the boiling water. Allow for a 10-min rest period after covering. Using a fork, fluff the mixture.
4. Toss the couscous, cherry tomatoes, cucumber, artichoke hearts, avocado, and pine nuts together in a large mixing basin. Toss in the dressing to mix. Serve after 1 hour in the refrigerator.

Nutrition: Calories: 489 Fat: 30g Carbs: 46g Protein: 11g

5.20 Paprika Cauliflower Steaks with Walnut Sauce

Prep Time: 15 mins

Cook Time: 30 mins

Servings: 2

Ingredients:

- Walnut Sauce:
- ½ cup raw walnut halves
- 2 tbsp virgin olive oil, divided
- 1 clove garlic, chopped
- 1 small yellow onion, chopped
- ½ cup unsweetened almond milk
- 2 tbsp fresh lemon juice
- Salt and pepper, to taste
- Paprika Cauliflower:
- 1 medium head cauliflower
- 1 tsp sweet paprika

- 1 tsp minced fresh thyme leaves (about 2 sprigs)

Directions:

1. Preheat your oven to around 350 degrees Fahrenheit (180 degrees Celsius). To make the walnut sauce, follow these steps: 5 mins over medium heat, toast the walnuts in a large, ovenproof pan until fragrant and slightly browned. Place the walnuts in a blender and mix until smooth.
2. In a skillet, heat 1 tbsp of olive oil. Sauté for about 2 mins, or until the garlic and onion are slightly softened.
3. Combine the garlic and onion and the almond milk, lemon juice, salt, and pepper in a blender. Blend until the mixture is smooth and creamy. While you're preparing the cauliflower, keep the sauce warm.
4. To make the paprika cauliflower, follow these steps: Cut two 1-inch thick "steaks" from the cauliflower's middle. Season the steaks on both sides with paprika, thyme, salt, and pepper after lightly moistening them with water.
5. Heat the remaining 1 tbsp of olive oil in the same skillet over medium-high heat. Sear the cauliflower steaks for approximately 3 mins, or until they are uniformly browned. Transfer the pan to the oven after flipping the cauliflower steaks.
6. Roast for 20 mins in a preheated oven until crisp-tender. Warm cauliflower steaks are served with a side of walnut sauce.

Nutrition: Calories: 367 Fat: 27.9g Protein: 7.0g Carbs: 22.7g

5.21 Stir-Fried Eggplant

Prep Time: 15 mins

Cook Time: 15 mins

Servings: 2

Ingredients:

- 1 cup water, plus more as needed
- ½ cup chopped red onion
- 1 tbsp finely chopped garlic
- 1 tbsp dried Italian herb seasoning
- 1 tsp ground cumin
- 1 small eggplant (about 8 oz / 227 g), peeled and cut into ½-inch cubes
- 1 medium carrot, sliced
- 2 cups pinto beans, cut into 1-inch pieces
- 2 ribs celery, sliced
- 1 cup corn kernels
- 2 tbsp almond butter
- 2 medium tomatoes, chopped

Directions:

1. Boil 1 tbsp of water over medium-high heat until it sputters in a large soup pot. Cook for 2 mins, adding a splash of water if necessary.
2. Stir-fry for 2 to 3 mins with the garlic, Italian seasoning, cumin, and eggplant, adding a little more water as required.
3. Stir in the carrots, pinto beans, celery, corn kernels, and 12 cups water. Reduce the heat to medium, cover, and simmer for 8 to 10 mins, or until the veggies are soft, stirring occasionally. Meanwhile, combine the almond butter and 12 cups of water in a mixing dish.
4. Stir in the almond butter mixture and chopped tomatoes after removing the veggies from the heat. Before serving, let it cool for a few mins.

Nutrition: Calories: 176 Fat: 5.5g Protein: 5.8g Carbs: 25.4g

5.22 Pad Thai

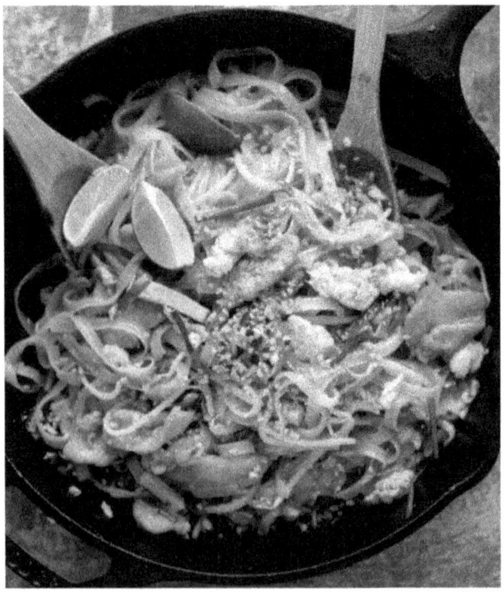

Prep Time: 15 mins

Cook Time: 15 mins

Servings: 2

Ingredients:

- 1 diced shallot
- 2 tbsp of peanut oil
- 4 minced garlic cloves
- salt and pepper to taste
- 4 oz. of pad thai noodles
- 1 tsp of chopped ginger
- 6 to 8 oz. tofu
- 1 lime

Sauce:

- 1 tsp of gluten-free liquid aminos
- 3 tbsp of brown sugar
- 3 tbsp of vegan fish sauce
- 3 tbsp of rice vinegar

Directions:

1. Cook the noodles according to the package directions.
2. Whisk together all the sauce's ingredients in a mixing bowl.
3. Season the tofu cubes with salt and pepper. Cook for 4-5 mins in a little amount of heated oil before transferring to a platter.
4. Sauté ginger, shallot, and garlic in heated oil for 2-3 mins in a wok.
5. Toss in the noodles, cooked tofu, and other ingredients until well heated.
6. Serve.

Nutrition: Calories: 575 Fat: 23.5g Protein: 2.8g Carbs: 90.6g

5.23 Quick Steamed Broccoli

Prep Time: 15 mins

Cook Time: 5 mins

Servings: 2

Ingredients:

- ¼ cup water
- 3 cups broccoli florets
- Salt and ground black pepper, to taste

Directions:

1. Fill the deep pot halfway with water. Fill the pot halfway with broccoli florets.
2. Put the cover back on. Cook for roughly 5 mins on high heat. Open the lid with care.
3. To retain the beautiful green color of the broccoli florets, place them in a dish with cold water. Season the broccoli to taste with salt and pepper before serving.

Nutrition: Calories: 16 Fat: 0.2g Protein: 1.9g Carbs: 1.7g

5.24 Tempeh Lettuce Wraps

Prep Time: 20 Mins

Cook Time: 15 Mins

Servings: 4

Ingredients:

- 1 cup of vegetable broth
- 1/4 tsp of ground coriander
- 1 tsp of gluten-free tamari
- 8 oz of tempeh
- 1/4 cups of red cabbage, sliced thin
- 8 leaves of butter lettuce
- 1 tsp of maple syrup
- 1/8 tsp of garlic powder
- 1 sliced red bell pepper
- 1 peeled carrot, julienned
- Peanut sauce, for serving

Directions:

1 Add the broken tempeh to a food processor and pulse until it crumbles.

2 Lettuce, veggies, and tempeh, combine the other ingredients in a mixing bowl.

3 Combine the tempeh and the ingredients in a pan. Cook for 8-9 mins, stirring occasionally; even though it seems dry, it will contain some moisture.

4 When all the liquid has been absorbed, turn off the heat.

5 Place the veggies and tempeh in each lettuce wrap. Serve with a drizzle of peanut sauce and a bun.

Nutrition for 2 wraps: Calories: 201 Fat: 7.2 g Carbs: 23.6 g Protein: 2 g

5.25 Cucumber Salad with lemon

Prep Time: 10 mins

Cook Time: 10 mins

Servings: 6

Ingredients:

- For salad:
- ¼ cup fresh basil leaves, chopped
- ¼ cup fresh mint leaves, chopped
- 1 cucumber, cubed
- For dressing:
- 1 tbsp olive oil - 2 tbsp fresh lime juice
- Pinch of salt

Directions:

1. Combine all dressing ingredients in a small dish and put it aside. In a mixing basin, combine all salad ingredients and stir thoroughly.
2. Toss the salad thoroughly with the dressing. Serve and have fun.

Nutrition: Calories: 130 Fat: 7.6g Protein: 3.5g Carbs: 13.9g

5.26 Potatoes with Lemon Kale & White Beans

Prep Time: 15 Mins

Cook Time: 60 Mins

Servings: 2-4

Ingredients:

- 1 tbsp of olive oil
- 1 to 2 minced garlic cloves

- 4 sweet potatoes
- Half-1 tsp of red pepper flakes
- 1 tsp of lemon zest
- sea salt, to taste
- 1 bunch of kale, chopped without thick stems
- 1 chopped shallot
- Half a lemon's juice
- 1 can of (15 oz) Cannellini beans

Directions:

1. Preheat your oven to around 350 degrees Fahrenheit.
2. Prick the sweet potato all over with a fork and bake for 45-60 mins, until tender.
3. Heat the oil in a skillet and cook the shallots for 2 mins.
4. Cook for 60 seconds after adding the lemon zest, garlic, and salt.
5. Cook for 2-3 mins after adding the beans, pepper flakes, and greens.
6. Adjust the flavor with lemon juice. Turn off the heat.
7. Allow the sweet potatoes to cool slightly before cutting them in half and topping with the remaining mixture.
8. Serve.

Nutrition: Calories: 295 Fat: 8.5 g Carbs: 46 g Protein: 12 g

5.27 Creamy Kale and Mushrooms

Prep Time: 15 mins

Cook Time: 15 mins

Servings: 3

Ingredients:

- 3 tbsp coconut oil
- 3 cloves of garlic, minced
- 1 onion, chopped
- 1 bunch kale, stems removed and leaves chopped
- 5 white button mushrooms, chopped
- 1 cup of coconut milk
- Salt and pepper to taste

Directions:

1. In a saucepan, heat the oil. For 2 mins, sauté the garlic and onion until aromatic. Add the mushrooms and mix well. Season with salt and pepper. Cook for a further 8 mins.
2. Combine the greens and coconut milk in a mixing bowl. Cook for 5 mins on low heat. Season with salt and pepper to taste.

Nutrition: Calories: 365 Fat: 33.5 g Carbs: 17.9 g Protein: 6 g

5.28 Mediterranean Cauliflower Rice

Prep Time: 15 Mins

Cook Time: 15 Mins

Servings: 2-3

Ingredients:

- 1/4 tsp of red chili flakes
- 1/4 cup of diced onion
- 3 cups riced cauliflower
- half lemon's zest
- 1 tbsp of olive oil
- 2 minced garlic cloves
- 1 tbsp of lemon juice
- 2 tbsp of pine nuts

Directions:

1 For 4-5 mins, sauté onion in heated oil.

2 Cook for 1-2 mins after adding the garlic.

3 Increase the heat to high and add the chili flakes, cauliflower, pine nuts, lemon zest, and juice. Cook for 1 min or until desired consistency is reached.

4 Remove the pan from the heat and stir in the parsley. Season with salt and pepper to taste, then serve.

5 Remove the pan from the heat and whisk in the parsley. Then season to taste with salt and pepper and serve.

Nutrition: Calories: 216 Fat: 3 g Carbs: 8 g Protein: 5 g

5.29 Sautéed Dark Leafy Greens

Prep Time: 15 mins

Cook Time: 10 mins

Servings: 4

Ingredients:

- 2 tbsp olive oil
- 8 cups stemmed and coarsely chopped spinach, kale, collard greens, or Swiss chard
- Juice of ½ lemon
- Sea salt
- Freshly ground black pepper

Directions:

1. Heat the olive oil in a large pan over medium-high heat. Toss the greens with tongs until they are wilted and soft, about 8 to 10 mins.

2. Remove the pan from the heat and add the lemon juice, swirling to cover all vegetables uniformly. Serve with a pinch of salt and pepper.

Nutrition: Calories: 129 Fat: 7g Carbs: 14g Protein: 8 g

5.30 Tomato salad with olive oil

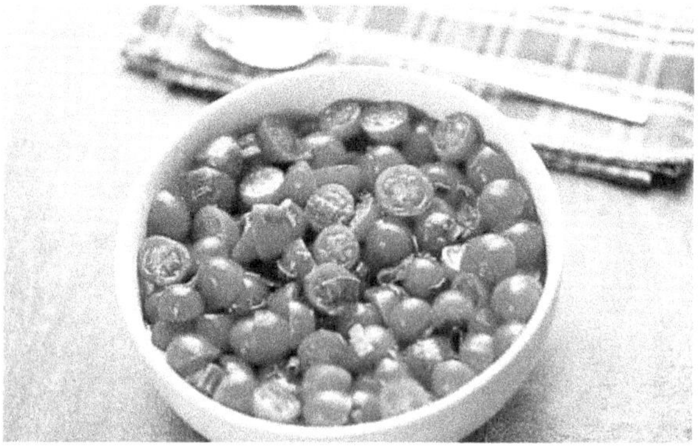

Prep Time: 15 mins

Cook Time: 8 mins

Servings: 4

Ingredients:

- 4 large tomatoes, cut in half horizontally
- 1 tbsp olive oil
- 1 tsp minced garlic
- 1 tbsp chopped fresh basil
- Sea salt
- Freshly ground black pepper

Directions:

1. Preheat the broiler in the oven. Drizzle the olive oil over the tomato halves, cut-side up, in a 9-by-13-inch baking dish. Garlic should be rubbed into the tomatoes.
2. Broil for approximately 5 mins, or until the tomatoes are softened. Season with salt & pepper and a pinch of basil. Serve.

Nutrition: Calories: 113 Fat: 8g Carbs: 8g Protein: 4g

5.31 Wild Rice with Grapes

Prep Time: 15 mins

Cook Time: 50 mins

Servings: 4

Ingredients:

- 1 cup wild rice blend
- 1¾ cups water
- 1 tsp olive oil
- 2 cups red seedless grapes
- 2 tsp chopped fresh thyme
- Sea salt
- Freshly ground black pepper

Directions:

1. Bring the rice, water, and salt to a boil in a saucepan. Cover, turn to low heat, and cook for 45 mins. Remove from the heat and set aside for 10 mins, covered. Using a fork, fluff the mixture.
2. Heat the olive oil in a large pan over medium-high heat. Sauté the grapes and thyme together for approximately 5 mins, or until the grapes begin to burst. Season with salt and pepper and stir in the wild rice mixture. Serve.

Nutrition: Calories: 146 Fat: 2g Carbs: 31g Protein: 3g

5.32 Traditional Falafel

Prep Time: 15 mins

Cook Time: 10 mins

Servings: 4

Ingredients:

- 1 (15-oz) can low-sodium chickpeas, drained and rinsed
- ½ sweet onion, chopped
- ¼ cup whole-wheat flour
- ¼ cup coarsely chopped fresh parsley
- ¼ cup coarsely chopped fresh cilantro
- Juice from 1 lemon
- 1 tbsp minced garlic
- 2 tsp ground cumin
- Sea salt
- Freshly ground black pepper
- 2 tbsp olive oil

Directions:

1. Stir the chickpeas, onion, flour, parsley, cilantro, lemon juice, garlic, and cumin in a food processor until the mixture barely holds together. Season with salt and pepper, then toss one more.
2. Scoop approximately 2 tsp of the mixture into a ball, shape it into a thick patty, and flatten it slightly. Carry on with the rest of the chickpea mixture.
3. Heat the olive oil in a large skillet over medium-high heat and pan-fry the patties until golden brown on both sides, approximately 4 mins each side. Serve on its own or in pita bread.

Nutrition: Calories: 245 Fat: 9g Carbs: 36g Protein: 7g

5.33 Spicy Split Pea Tabbouleh

Prep Time: 1 hour & 15 mins

Cook Time: 45 mins

Servings: 6

Ingredients:

- 1½ cups split peas
- 4 cups water
- 2 large tomatoes, seeded and chopped
- 1 English cucumber, chopped
- 1 yellow bell pepper, chopped
- 1 orange bell pepper, chopped
- ½ red onion, finely chopped
- ¼ cup chopped fresh cilantro
- Juice of 1 lime
- 1 tsp ground cumin
- ½ tsp ground coriander
- Pinch red pepper flakes
- Sea salt
- Freshly ground black pepper

Directions:

1. Bring the split peas and water to a boil in a large saucepan over medium-high heat. Reduce the heat to low and cook, uncovered, for 40 to 45 mins, or until the peas are soft. Drain the peas and chill them by rinsing them in cold water.
2. Toss the peas with the tomatoes, cucumber, bell peppers, onion, cilantro, lime juice, cumin, coriander, and red pepper flakes in a large mixing dish. Toss well to combine.
3. Refrigerate the mixture for at least 1 hour to allow the flavors to meld. Serve with a pinch of salt and pepper.

Nutrition: Calories: 208 Fat: 1g Carbs: 38g Protein: 14g

5.34 Mashed Avocado with fresh parsley

Prep Time: 15 mins

Cook Time: 0 mins

Servings: 4

Ingredients:

- 1 avocado, peeled and pitted
- 1 celery stalk, chopped
- Juice and zest of ½ lemon
- 1 tsp chopped fresh parsley
- 4 whole-wheat bread slices, toasted
- 2 tomatoes, thinly sliced
- Sea salt
- Freshly ground black pepper

Directions:

1. Mash the avocado in a medium bowl until smooth but slightly lumpy. Combine the celery, lemon juice, lemon zest, and parsley in a large mixing bowl.
2. Spread the mixture generously over the bread and top with tomato slices. Serve with a pinch of salt and pepper.

Nutrition: Calories: 248 Fat: 14g Carbs: 18g Protein: 13g

5.35 Sweet Potato & Brussel Sprout Vegan Tacos

Prep Time: 15 Mins

Cook Time: 20 Mins

Servings: 8

Ingredients:

- 3 tbsp of olive oil
- Half diced yellow onion
- 1 lb. of peeled & cubed sweet potatoes
- 1 diced green bell pepper
- gluten-free tortillas
- 2 crushed garlic cloves
- 1 tsp of salt
- 1 lb. of sliced Brussel sprouts
- 2 tsp of apple cider vinegar
- 1 tsp of hot sauce
- 2 tbsp of maple syrup
- ¼ tsp of ground sage

Directions:

1 Heat the oil in a pan and cook the onion and bell pepper for 2-3 mins.

2 Cook for 6 to 8 mins after adding the sweet potatoes.

3 Cook for 3 to 4 mins, covered with sprouts.

4 Mix the other ingredients in a bowl, except the tortillas. Cook for 2 to 3 mins after adding to the pan.

5 Place the mixture in each tortilla and serve.

Nutrition: Calories: 283 Fat: 13 g Carbs: 39 g Protein: 3 g

5.36 Mediterranean Brussels Sprouts

Prep Time: 15 mins

Cook Time: 23 mins

Servings: 4

Ingredients:

- 2 cups Brussels sprouts, cut in half
- ¼ cup olive oil

- 1 bay leaf - 2 tsp pine nuts, roasted
- ½ cup olives
- 2 tbsp sun-dried tomatoes, chopped
- Pepper - Salt

Directions:

1. Preheat your oven to around 3500 degrees Fahrenheit. In a medium-sized pan, heat 1 tbsp of oil. Cook for 7-8 mins with Brussels sprouts and salt. Preheat your oven to around 350°F and roast the sprouts for 10 mins.
2. Meanwhile, heat the remaining oil in a separate pan over medium heat. Cook for 5 mins after adding the sun-dried tomatoes and olives.
3. Take the sprouts out of the oven and combine them with the tomato-olive mixture. Serve with pine nuts on top.

Nutrition: Calories: 182 Fat: 17.5 g Carbs: 5.9 g Protein: 3.2 g

5.37 Eggplant with Italian seasoning

Prep Time: 15 mins

Cook Time: 10 mins

Servings: 4

Ingredients:

- 1 eggplant, cut into 1-inch pieces
- ½ cup of water
- ¼ cup Can tomato, crushed
- ½ tsp Italian seasoning
- 1 tsp paprika - ½ tsp chili powder
- 1 tsp garlic powder
- 2 tbsp olive oil - Salt

Directions:

1. Fill the deep saucepan halfway with water and the eggplant. Cook on high for 5 mins after sealing the pot with a cover.
2. Clean the saucepan after draining the eggplant. Fill the saucepan with oil.
3. Stir in the eggplant and the additional ingredients, and simmer for 5 mins. Serve and have fun.

Nutrition: Calories: 97 Fat: 7.5 g Carbs: 8.2 g Protein: 1.5 g

5.38 Indian Bell Peppers and Potato Stir Fry

Prep Time: 15 mins

Cook Time: 10 mins

Servings: 2

Ingredients:

- 1 tbsp oil
- ½ tsp cumin seeds
- 4 cloves of garlic, minced
- 4 potatoes, scrubbed and halved
- Salt and pepper to taste
- 5 tbsp water
- 2 bell peppers, seeded and julienned
- Chopped cilantro for garnish

Directions:

1. In a medium-sized pan, heat the oil and roast the cumin seeds until fragrant. Add the garlic and cook until it is fragrant. Combine the potatoes, salt, pepper, water, and bell peppers in a large mixing bowl.
2. Allow boiling for at least 10 mins with the lid closed. Before the cooking time is up, garnish with cilantro. Place each item in its container.
3. Put a label on it and put it in the refrigerator. Allow for room temperature thawing before heating in the microwave.

Nutrition: Calories: 83 Fat: 6.4 g Carbs: 7.3 g Protein: 2.8 g

5.39 Carrot Potato with chopped onion

Prep Time: 15 mins

Cook Time: 15 mins

Servings: 6

Ingredients:

- 4 lbs. Baby potatoes, clean and cut in half
- 1 ½ lb. Carrots, cut into chunks
- 1 tsp Italian seasoning
- 1 ½ cups vegetable broth
- 1 tbsp garlic, chopped
- 1 onion, chopped
- 2 tbsp olive oil
- Pepper
- Salt

Directions:

1. In a big saucepan, pour in the oil. Cook for 5 mins after adding the onion. Cook for 5 mins after adding the carrots.
2. Stir in the remaining ingredients well. Cook for 5 mins on high with the cover on the pot.
3. Take off the cover. Serve after a quick stir.

Nutrition: Calories: 283 Fat: 5.6 g Carbs: 51.3 g Protein: 10.2 g

5.40 Potatoes with paprika

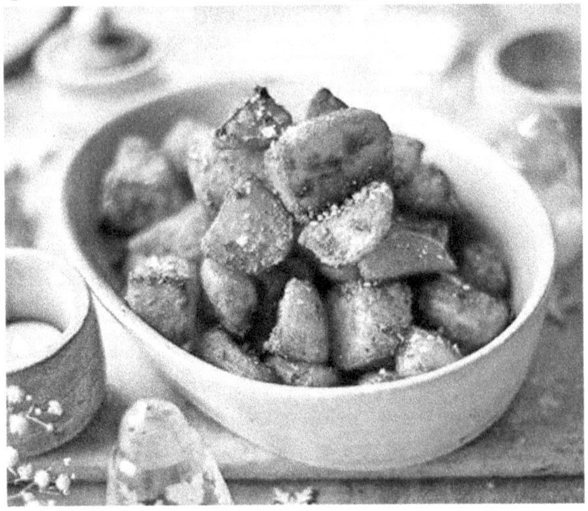

Prep Time: 15 mins

Cook Time: 35 mins

Servings: 8

Ingredients:

- 4 large, sweet potatoes, peel, and cut into 1-inch cubes
- ¼ tsp paprika
- 2 tbsp olive oil
- 8 sage leaves
- 2 tsp vinegar
- ½ tsp of sea salt

Directions:

1. Preheat the oven to 375 degrees Fahrenheit. Combine the sweet potato, olive oil, sage, and salt in a large mixing basin. Toss thoroughly. 35 mins in the oven
2. Mix in the vinegar and paprika well. Serve and have fun.

Nutrition: Calories: 90 Fat: 3.5 g Carbs: 14 g Protein: 1 g

5.41 Eggplant with fresh basil

Prep Time: 15 mins

Cook Time: 10 mins

Servings: 8

Ingredients:

- 1 small eggplant, cut into cubes
- 1 cup fresh basil
- 2 cups grape tomatoes
- 1 onion, chopped
- 2 summer squash, sliced
- 2 zucchinis, sliced
- 2 tbsp vinegar
- 2 tbsp tomato paste
- 1 tbsp garlic, minced
- 1 fresh lemon juice
- ¼ cup olive oil
- Salt

Directions:

1. In a blender, combine the basil, vinegar, tomato paste, garlic, lemon juice, oil, and salt until smooth. Combine the eggplant, tomatoes, onion, squash, and zucchini in a saucepan.
2. Pour the basil mixture over the veggies and stir well. Cook for 10 mins on high with the lid on the pot. Take off the cover. Serve with a good stir.

Nutrition: Calories: 103 Fat: 6.8 g Carbs: 10.6 g Protein: 2.4 g

5.42 Roasted Vinegar Cauliflower

Prep Time: 15 mins

Cook Time: 30 mins

Servings: 4

Ingredients:

- 8 cups cauliflower florets
- 1 tsp dried marjoram
- 2 tbsp olive oil
- 2 tbsp vinegar
- ¼ tsp pepper
- ¼ tsp salt

Directions:

1. Preheat the oven to 450 degrees Fahrenheit. Combine the cauliflower, marjoram, oil, pepper, and salt in a mixing bowl. Toss thoroughly. Roast the cauliflower for 15-20 mins after spreading it out on the oven dish.
2. Combine the cauliflower and the vinegar in a mixing bowl. Return the cauliflower to the oven for another 5-10 mins of roasting. Serve and have fun.

Nutrition: Calories: 196 Fat: 13 g Carbs: 11 g Protein: 11 g

5.43 Cauliflower Walnut Taco Meat

Prep Time: 20 Mins

Cook Time: 30 Mins

Servings: 6-8

Ingredients:

Taco Meat:

- 12 oz. of cauliflower florets
- 1 cup of walnuts
- 2 tbsp of nutritional yeast
- to 10 oz. button mushrooms, sliced
- 2 tsp of olive oil

Spice Mixture:

- 2 tsp of chili powder
- 3/4 tsp of cumin
- 1 tsp of dried oregano
- 1 tsp of garlic powder
- 1 tbsp of coconut sugar
- 2 1/2 tsp of smoked paprika
- 1 1/2 tsp of onion powder
- Sea salt & black pepper, to taste

Directions:

1 Preheat your oven to around 350 degrees Fahrenheit. On a baking pan, toast the walnuts for 8-10 mins.
2 Put them in a bowl and preheat the oven to 400 degrees Fahrenheit.
3 Toss the mushroom and cauliflower with the oil on a parchment-lined baking pan.
4 20 mins of roasting
5 Pulse the spice combination (1/4 cup), yeast, and walnuts until barely incorporated in a food processor.
6 Pulse the roasted veggies until they are barely blended in the food processor.
7 Season to taste with the spice combination.
8 Serve with gluten-free rice or tortillas.

Nutrition: Calories: 234 Fat: 8 g Carbs: 4 g Protein: 6 g

5.44 Brussels Sprouts with Cranberries

Prep Time: 15 mins

Cook Time: 10 mins

Servings: 6

Ingredients:

- 1 lb. Brussels sprouts, cut in half
- ½ cup dried cranberries
- ½ pecans, toasted
- 1 tbsp vinegar
- 3 tbsp olive oil
- Pepper
- Salt

Directions:

1. In a pan over medium-high heat, heat the oil. Cook for 5 mins after adding the Brussels sprouts. Cook for another 5 mins after seasoning with pepper and salt.
2. Drizzle in the vinegar and give it a good swirl. Turn off the heat in the pan. Toss the Brussels sprouts with the pecans and cranberries in a large mixing basin. Serve and have fun.

Nutrition: Calories: 170 Fat: 13.8 g Carbs: 8.7 g Protein: 5.5 g

5.45 Asparagus Salad with lemon

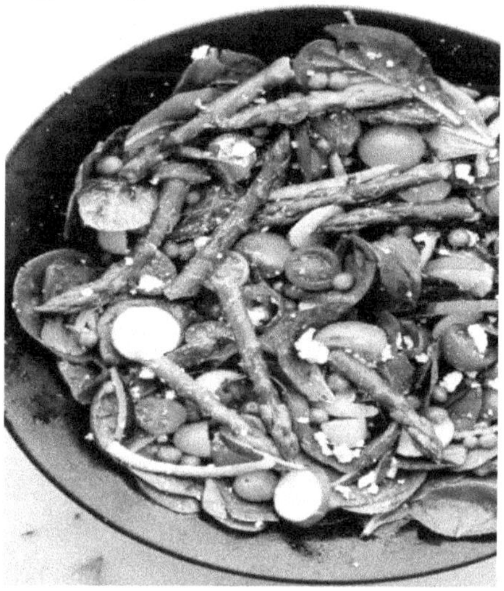

Prep Time: 10 mins

Cook Time: 10 mins

Servings: 4

Ingredients:

- 2 lb. Asparagus, ends trimmed
- 1 tbsp. lemon juice
- 1 lemon zest
- 3 tbsp olive oil
- ¼ tsp pepper
- ¼ tsp salt

Directions:

1. Preheat the grill to a high temperature. Arrange asparagus on a baking sheet coated with foil. Season with pepper and salt and drizzle with 2 tbsp of oil.
2. Cook the asparagus for 3-4 mins on the grill. Transfer the grilled asparagus to a mixing bowl and chop it up.
3. Toss in the remaining ingredients in the mixing bowl. Serve and have fun.

Nutrition: Calories: 211 Fat: 16.8g Protein: 9g Carbs: 10.1g

CHAPTER 6:

Fish & Seafood

6.1 Fast Seafood Paella

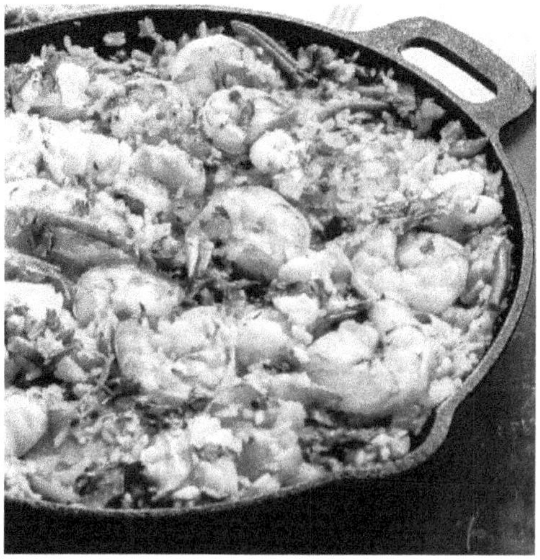

Prep Time: 15 mins

Cook Time: 20 mins

Servings: 4

Ingredients:

- ¼ cup plus 1 tbsp extra-virgin olive oil
- 1 large onion, finely chopped
- 2 tomatoes, peeled and chopped
- 1½ tbsp garlic powder
- 1½ cups medium-grain Spanish paella rice or arborio rice
- 2 carrots, finely diced
- Salt, to taste
- 1 tbsp sweet paprika
- 8 oz (227 g) lobster meat or canned crab
- ½ cup frozen peas
- 3 cups chicken stock, plus more if needed
- 1 cup dry white wine
- 6 jumbo shrimp, unpeeled
- 1/3-pound (136 g) calamari rings
- 1 lemon, halved

Directions:

1. Heat the oil in a big sauté pan or skillet (16-inch is excellent) over medium heat until little bubbles emerge.
2. Cook for approximately 3 mins until the onion is aromatic, then add the tomatoes and garlic powder. Cook for 5 to 10 mins, or until the tomatoes have been reduced by half and the sauce has thickened to a sticky consistency.
3. Combine the rice, carrots, salt, paprika, lobster, and peas in a large mixing bowl. Heat the chicken stock to nearly boiling in a saucepan or microwave-safe dish before adding it to the rice mixture. Bring to a low simmer before adding the wine.
4. Smooth out the rice in the pan's bottom. Cover and simmer on low for 10 mins to avoid burning, stirring regularly.
5. Cover and simmer for another 5 mins after adding the shrimp to the rice. If the rice seems to be dry, add more liquid to the pan.
6. Add the calamari rings just before taking the pan off the heat. Frequently toss the ingredients.
7. The rings will become opaque after approximately 2 mins. Remove the pan from the heat as soon as possible to avoid overcooking the paella). Fresh lemon juice should be squeezed over the meal.

Nutrition: Calories: 632 Fat: 20g Protein: 34g Carbs: 71g

6.2 Crispy Fried Sardines

Prep Time: 15 mins

Cook Time: 5 mins

Servings: 4

Ingredients:

- Avocado oil, as needed
- 1½ pounds (680 g) whole fresh sardines, scales removed
- 1 tsp salt
- 1 tsp freshly ground black pepper
- 2 cups flour

Directions:

1. Preheat a heavy-bottomed skillet over medium-high heat. Pour in enough oil to cover the bottom of the pan by approximately 1 inch. Season the fish with salt and pepper before serving.

2. Using the flour, dredge the fish until it is thoroughly coated. Drop 1 fish at a time into the pan, being careful not to overcrowd it.
3. Cook for 3 mins on each side, or until the salmon is golden brown on both sides. Warm the dish before serving.

Nutrition: Calories: 794 Fat: 47g Protein: 48g Carbs: 44g

6.3 Orange Roasted Salmon

Prep Time: 15 mins

Cook Time: 25 mins

Servings: 4

Ingredients:

- ½ cup extra-virgin olive oil, divided
- 2 tbsp balsamic vinegar
- 2 tbsp garlic powder, divided
- 1 tbsp cumin seeds
- 1 tsp sea salt, divided
- 1 tsp freshly ground black pepper, divided
- 2 tsp smoked paprika
- 4 (8-oz / 227-g) wild salmon fillets, skinless
- 2 small red onions, thinly sliced
- ½ cup halved Campari tomatoes
- 1 small fennel bulb, thinly sliced lengthwise
- 1 large carrot, thinly sliced
- 8 medium portobello mushrooms
- 8 medium radishes, sliced 1/8 inch thick
- ½ cup dry white wine
- ½ lime, zested
- Handful cilantro leaves
- ½ cup halved pitted Kalamata olives
- 1 orange, thinly sliced
- 4 roasted sweet potatoes, cut in wedges lengthwise

Directions:

1. Preheat the oven to 375 degrees Fahrenheit (190 degrees Celsius). 6 tbsp olive oil, 1 tbsp balsamic vinegar, 1 tbsp garlic powder, cumin seeds, 14 tsp sea salt, 14 tsp pepper, and paprika in a medium bowl
2. Place the salmon in a basin and marinate for 10 minutes while preparing the veggies.
3. Sear the top of the salmon for approximately 2 mins, or until nicely browned, in an oven-safe sauté pan or skillet over medium-high heat. Remove from the equation.
4. In the same skillet, add the remaining 2 tbsp of olive oil. Add the onion, tomatoes, fennel, carrot, mushrooms, radishes, 1 tsp garlic powder, 34 tsp salt, and 34 tsp pepper once it's heated.
5. Cook, constantly stirring, for 5 to 7 mins, or until aromatic. Mix in the wine well. Place the browned-side-up salmon on top of the veggie mixture.
6. Place the olives around the fish and sprinkle it with lime zest and cilantro. Cook for a further 7 mins after adding the orange slices to the fish.
7. Add the cut sweet potato wedges on a baking sheet and roast beside the skillet while it bakes. Remove the pan from the oven, cover securely, and set aside for 3 mins.

Nutrition: Calories: 841 Fat: 41g Protein: 59g Carbs: 60g

6.4 Lemon Rosemary Branzino

Prep Time: 15 mins

Cook Time: 30 mins

Servings: 4

Ingredients:

- 4 tbsp extra-virgin olive oil, divided
- 2 (8-oz / 227-g) branzino fillets, preferably at least 1 inch thick
- 1 garlic clove, minced
- 1 bunch scallions, white part only, thinly sliced
- ½ cup sliced pitted Kalamata or other good-quality black olives
- 1 large carrot, cut into ¼-inch rounds
- 10 to 12 small cherry tomatoes, halved
- ½ cup dry white wine
- 2 tbsp paprika
- 2 tsp kosher salt
- ½ tbsp ground chili pepper, preferably Turkish or Aleppo
- 2 rosemary sprigs or 1 tbsp dried rosemary
- 1 small lemon, very thinly sliced

Directions:

1. Warm a big, oven-safe sauté pan or skillet for 2 mins over high heat. 1 tbsp olive oil, carefully added and heated until it shimmers, 10 to 15 seconds
2. Brown the branzino fillets skin-side up for 2 mins. Cook for another 2 mins until the fillets are browned on the skin side. Remove from the equation.
3. 2 tbsp olive oil, swirled around the pan to evenly coat it. Add the garlic, scallions, kalamata olives, carrots, and tomatoes and

cook for 5 mins, or until the veggies have softened.

4. Stir in the wine until all the ingredients are fully combined. Place the fish on top of the sauce with care. Preheat the oven to 450 degrees Fahrenheit (235 degrees Celsius).
5. Brush the fillets with 1 tbsp olive oil and season with paprika, salt, and chili pepper while the oven is heating up.
6. A rosemary sprig and several lemon slices should be placed on each fillet. Arrange the olives on top of the fish and around the pan. Roast for approximately 10 mins, or until the lemon slices are browned or roasted.

Nutrition: calories: 725 Fat: 43g protein: 58g carbs: 25g

6.5 Almond-Crusted Swordfish

Prep Time: 15 mins

Cook Time: 15 mins

Servings: 4

Ingredients:

- ½ cup almond flour
- ¼ cup crushed Marcona almonds
- ½ to 1 tsp salt, divided
- 2 pounds (907 g) Swordfish, preferably 1 inch thick
- 1 large egg, beaten (optional)
- ¼ cup pure apple cider
- ¼ cup extra-virgin olive oil, plus more for frying
- 3 to 4 sprigs flat-leaf parsley, chopped
- 1 lemon, juiced
- 1 tbsp Spanish paprika
- 5 medium baby portobello mushrooms, chopped (optional)
- 4 or 5 chopped scallions, both green and white parts
- 3 to 4 garlic cloves, peeled
- ¼ cup chopped pitted Kalamata olives

Directions:

1. Spread the flour and crushed Marcona almonds on a dinner plate and season with salt. Fill a big plastic food storage bag halfway with flour, nuts, and 14 tsp of salt.
2. Add the fish to the flour mixture and coat it well. If you want a thicker covering, repeat the process after dipping the fish in the egg (if using).
3. Combine the apple cider, 14 cups olive oil, parsley, lemon juice, paprika, and 14 tsp salt in a measuring cup. Set aside after thoroughly mixing.
4. Pour the olive oil to a depth of 18 inches in a big, heavy-bottomed sauté pan or skillet and heat over medium heat.
5. When the oil is heated, add the fish, and cook for 3 to 5 mins, then flip the fish and add the mushrooms, onions, garlic, and olives (if using).
6. Cook for a further 3 mins. Remove the fish from the pan after the other side is brown and put it aside.
7. Pour the cider mixture into the pan with the veggies and stir thoroughly. Place the fried fish on top of the mixture in the pan and cook for 10 mins over medium-low heat until the fish flakes easily with a fork.
8. Remove the fish from the pan with care and place it on a platter. Using a spoon, drizzle the sauce over the fish. Serve with white rice or fried potatoes from scratch.

Nutrition: Calories: 620 Fat: 37g Protein: 63g Carbs: 10g

6.6 Sea Bass Crusted with Moroccan Spices

Prep Time: 15 mins

Cook Time: 40 mins

Servings: 4

Ingredients:

- 1½ tsp ground turmeric, divided
- ¾ tsp saffron
- ½ tsp ground cumin
- ¼ tsp kosher salt
- ¼ tsp freshly ground black pepper
- 1½ pounds (680 g) sea bass fillets, about ½ inch thick
- 8 tbsp extra-virgin olive oil, divided
- 8 garlic cloves, divided (4 minced cloves and 4 sliced)
- 6 medium baby portobello mushrooms, chopped
- 1 large carrot, sliced at an angle
- 2 sun-dried tomatoes, thinly sliced (optional)
- 2 tbsp tomato paste
- 1 (15-oz / 425-g) can chickpeas, drained and rinsed
- 1½ cups low-sodium vegetable broth
- ¼ cup white wine
- 1 tbsp ground coriander (optional)
- 1 cup sliced artichoke hearts marinated in olive oil

- ½ cup pitted Kalamata olives
- ½ lemon, juiced
- ½ lemon, cut into thin rounds
- 4 to 5 rosemary sprigs or 2 tbsp dried rosemary
- Fresh cilantro, for garnish

Directions:

1. Combine 1 tsp turmeric, saffron, and cumin in a small mixing bowl. Salt and pepper to taste. The spice mixture should be applied to both sides of the fish.
2. 3 tbsp olive oil, worked into the fish to ensure it is fully covered in spices and olive oil.
3. 2 tsp olive oil, heated in a large sauté pan or skillet over medium heat until shimmering but not smoking. Sear the top side of the sea bass for 1 min or until golden brown. Remove the item and place it away.
4. Add the minced garlic to the same pan and simmer for a few mins, often stirring, until fragrant. Combine the mushrooms, carrots, sun-dried tomatoes (if using), and tomato paste in a large mixing bowl.
5. Cook, stirring regularly, for 3 to 4 mins over medium heat, until aromatic. Combine the chickpeas, broth, wine, coriander (if using), and sliced garlic in a large mixing bowl.
6. Add the remaining 12 tsp ground turmeric and mix well. If necessary, increase the heat to bring the mixture to a boil, then reduce to low heat to keep it simmering. Allow the sauce to boil, partially covered, for approximately 20 mins, or until thickened.
7. Add the seared fish to the skillet with care. Pour a little amount of the sauce over the fish. Combine the artichokes, olives, lemon juice and slices, and rosemary sprigs in a large mixing bowl.
8. Cook for another 10 mins, or until the fish is flaky and thoroughly cooked. Serve with fresh cilantro as a garnish.

Nutrition: Calories: 696 Fat: 41g Protein: 48g Carbs: 37g

6.7 Cilantro Lemon Shrimp

Prep Time: 20 mins

Cook Time: 10 mins

Servings: 4

Ingredients:

- 1/3 cup lemon juice
- 4 garlic cloves
- 1 cup fresh cilantro leaves
- ½ tsp ground coriander
- 3 tbsp extra-virgin olive oil
- 1 tsp salt
- 1½ pounds (680 g) large shrimp (21 to 25), deveined and shells removed

Directions:

1. Pulse the lemon juice, garlic, cilantro, coriander, olive oil, and salt 10 times in a food processor. Pour the cilantro marinade over the shrimp in a dish or plastic zip-top bag and set aside for 15 mins.
2. Warm a skillet over high heat. In a pan, combine the shrimp and marinade. Cook for 3 mins on each side of the shrimp. Warm the dish before serving.

Nutrition: Calories: 225 Fat: 12g Protein: 28g Carbs: 5g

6.8 Shrimp with Garlic and Mushrooms

Prep Time: 15 mins

Cook Time: 15 mins

Servings: 4

Ingredients:

- 1 pound (454 g) peeled and deveined fresh shrimp - 1 tsp salt
- 1 cup extra-virgin olive oil
- 8 large garlic cloves, thinly sliced
- 4 oz (113 g) sliced mushrooms (shiitake, baby Bella, or button)
- ½ tsp red pepper flakes
- ¼ cup chopped fresh flat-leaf Italian parsley
- Zucchini noodles or riced cauliflower, for serving

Directions:

1. Rinse and pat dry the shrimp. Place in a small mixing dish and season with salt. Heat the olive oil in a big rimmed, thick pan over medium-low heat.
2. Add the garlic and cook for 3 to 4 mins, or until extremely fragrant, lowering the heat if the garlic begins to burn.
3. Sauté the mushrooms for 5 mins, or until they are tender. Add the shrimp and red pepper flakes and cook for another 3 to 4 mins, or until the shrimp become pink.
4. Remove the pan from the heat and add the parsley. Serve over rice cauliflower or zucchini noodles.

Nutrition: Calories: 620 Fat: 56g Protein: 24g Carbs: 4g

6.9 Pistachio-Crusted Whitefish

Prep Time: 10 mins

Cook Time: 20 mins

Servings: 2

Ingredients:

- ¼ cup shelled pistachios
- 1 tbsp fresh parsley
- 1 tbsp panko breadcrumbs
- 2 tbsp olive oil
- ¼ tsp salt
- 10 oz' skinless whitefish (1 large piece or 2 smaller ones)

Directions:

1. Preheat your oven to around 350°F and place the center rack in the oven. Using foil or parchment paper, line a sheet pan.
2. In a tiny food processor, pulse all ingredients except the fish until the nuts are finely crushed.
3. Alternatively, you may use a chef's knife to mince the nuts and mix the ingredients in a small bowl by hand.
4. Place the fish on the baking sheet. Spread the nut mixture evenly on the fish and softly smooth it down.
5. Depending on the thickness of the fish, bake it for 20 to 30 mins, or until it flakes easily with a fork.
6. Remember that baking a thicker cut of fish takes a little longer. When it's opaque, flakes apart easily with a fork, or reaches an internal temperature of 145°F, you know it's done.

Nutrition: Calories: 185 Carbs: 23.8 g Protein: 10.1 g Fat: 5.2 g

6.10 Seafood Risotto

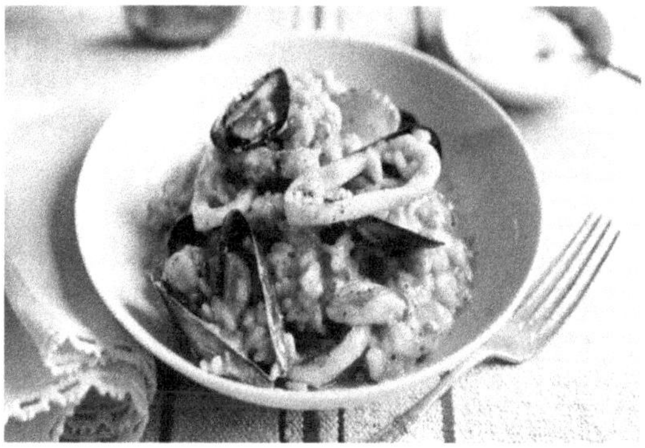

Prep Time: 15 mins

Cook Time: 30 mins

Servings: 4

Ingredients:

- 6 cups vegetable broth
- 3 tbsp extra-virgin olive oil
- 1 large onion, chopped
- 3 cloves minced garlic
- ½ tsp saffron threads
- 1½ cups arborio rice
- 1½ tsp salt
- 8 oz (227 g) shrimp (21 to 25), peeled and deveined
- 8 oz (227 g) scallops

Directions:

1. Bring the broth to a gentle boil in a big saucepan over medium heat. Cook the olive oil, onion, garlic, and saffron in a large pan on moderate heat for around 3 mins.
2. Combine the rice, salt, and 1 cup of stock in a pan. Combine the ingredients in a small saucepan and simmer over low heat until the liquid has almost evaporated.
3. Rep with broth, adding 12 cups at a time, and cooking until all except 12 cups of stock have been absorbed.
4. Add the shrimp and scallops when you whisk in the last 12 cups of broth. Cook for 10 mins with the lid on. Warm the dish before serving.

Nutrition: Calories: 460 Fat: 12g Protein: 24g Carbs: 64g

6.11 Crispy Homemade Fish Sticks Recipe

Prep Time: 10 mins

Cook Time: 15 mins

Servings: 2

Ingredients:

- ½ cup of flour
- 1 beaten egg
- 1 cup of flour
- ½ cup of breadcrumbs.
- Zest of 1 lemon juice
- Parsley
- Salt
- 1 tsp of black pepper
- 1 tbsp of sweet paprika
- 1 tsp of oregano
- 1 ½ lb. Of wild salmon
- Extra virgin olive oil

Directions:

1. Preheat the oven to 450 degrees Fahrenheit. Dry your fish in a basin and season both sides with salt.

2. Then slice into little pieces, each about 112 inches in length. In a bowl, combine black pepper and oregano.
3. Blend the paprika into the mixture. Then, season the fish stick using the spice mixture you just made. Pour the flours into a new dish.
4. You'll need a new basin to pour your egg wash into this time. Pick the fourth dish, combine the breadcrumbs and cheese, and stir in the lemon zest.
5. Return to the fish sticks and coat both sides of each one with flour. After dipping each fish in flour, remove it and dip it in an egg wash before finishing with the breadcrumb mixture.
6. Repeat with the remaining fish sticks and place them on a baking sheet. Oil the baking sheet before placing the fish sticks on it, then sprinkle extra virgin olive oil over the top of the fish sticks.
7. Allow extra flour from a fish to drip off before dipping it in additional ingredients.
8. Also, when adding extra virgin olive oil to the tops of the fish, make sure the coating does not peel.
9. Place the baking sheet in the center of the oven and bake for 13 mins. The fish should be golden brown by then, and you can remove them from the oven and serve right away.
10. Garnish with lemon zest, parsley, and freshly squeezed lemon juice.

Nutrition: Calories: 119 Fat: 3.4g Carbs: 9.3g Protein: 13.5g

6.12 Sauced Shellfish in White Wine

Prep Time: 10 mins

Cook Time: 10 mins

Servings: 2

Ingredients:

- 2-lbs fresh cuttlefish
- ½-cup olive oil
- 1-pc large onion, finely chopped
- 1-cup of Robola white wine
- ¼-cup lukewarm water
- 1-pc bay leaf
- ½-bunch parsley, chopped
- 4-pcs tomatoes, grated
- Salt and pepper

Directions:

1. Remove the cuttlefish's hard cartilage centerpiece (cuttlebone), the ink bag, and the guts.
2. Clean the cuttlefish under running water. Drain any extra water before slicing it into thin pieces.
3. In a medium-high-heat saucepan, heat the oil and sauté the onion for 3 mins or until tender.
4. Pour the white wine over the cuttlefish slices. Cook for 5 mins, or until it reaches a simmer.
5. After pouring in the water, add the tomatoes, bay leaf, parsley, tomatoes, salt, and pepper. Cook, occasionally stirring, until the cuttlefish pieces are cooked, and the sauce has thickened. Warm them up and serve with rice.
6. If you overcook the cuttlefish, the texture will become quite hard. Before using the cuttlefish in any dish, it's a good idea to grill it for 3 mins over a raging fire.

Nutrition: Calories: 308 Fat: 18.1g Carbs: 8g Protein: 25.6g

6.13 Pistachio Sole Fish

Prep Time: 5 mins

Cook Time: 10 mins

Servings: 2

Ingredients:

- 4 (5 oz) boneless sole fillets
- ½ cup pistachios, finely chopped
- Juice of 1 lemon
- Tsp extra virgin olive oil

Directions:

1. Preheat your oven to around 350 degrees Fahrenheit (180 degrees Celsius).
2. Wrap parchment paper around the baking sheet and set it aside.
3. Dry the fish with kitchen towels and season gently with salt and pepper.
4. Pistachios should be added to a small bowl.
5. Place the sol on the prepared sheet and top each fillet with 2 tsp of the pistachio mixture.
6. Lemon juice and olive oil are applied to the fish.
7. Bake for 10 mins, or until golden brown, and the fish flakes easily with a fork.

Nutrition: Calories: 166 Fat: 6g Carbs: 2g Protein 23g

6.14 Speedy Tilapia with Red Onion and Avocado

Prep Time: 10 mins

Cook Time: 5 mins

Servings: 2

Ingredients:

- 1 tbsp extra-virgin olive oil
- 1 tbsp freshly squeezed orange juice
- 1/4 tsp kosher or sea salt
- 4 (4-oz) tilapia fillets, more oblong than square, skin-on or skinned
- 1/4 cup chopped red onion (about 1/8 onion)
- 1 avocado, pitted, skinned, and sliced

Directions:

1. Mix the oil, orange juice, and salt with a fork in a 9-inch glass pie plate. Place each fish in the pie plate, one at a time, and flip to coat on both sides.
2. Arrange the fillets in a wagon-wheel pattern, with one end of each fillet in the middle of the dish and the other end draped over the dish's edge momentarily.
3. 1 tbsp onion on top of each fillet, then fold the end of the fillet that hangs over the edge in half over the onion.
4. When you're done, you should have four folded-over fillets with the fold against the dishes' outside edge and the ends all in the middle.
5. Wrap the dish with plastic wrap, leaving a tiny gap at the edge to allow steam to escape. Microwave for roughly 3 mins on high.
6. When gently prodded with a fork, the fish barely starts to split into flakes (chunks). Serve the fillets with avocado on top.

Nutrition: Carbs: 4 g Protein: 22 g Calories: 170 Fat: 8 g

6.15 Steamed Mussels in White Wine Sauce

Prep Time: 5 mins

Cook Time: 10 mins

Servings: 2

Ingredients:

- 2 pounds' small mussels
- 1 tbsp extra-virgin olive oil
- 1 cup thinly sliced red onion
- 3 garlic cloves, sliced
- 1 cup dry white wine
- 2 (1/4-inch-thick) lemon slices
- 1/4 tsp freshly ground black pepper
- 1/4 tsp kosher or sea salt
- Fresh lemon wedges, for serving (optional)

Directions:

1. Run cold water over the mussels in a big colander in the sink (but don't allow the mussels to stay in standing water).
2. All shells should be tightly closed; any slightly open or broken shells should be discarded. Remove the mussels from the colander and set them aside until ready to use.
3. Heat the oil in a large skillet over medium-high heat. Cook, stirring periodically, for 4 mins after adding the onion.
4. Cook, frequently stirring, for 1 min after adding the garlic. Bring the wine, lemon slices, pepper, and salt to a simmer in a saucepan. 2 mins in the oven
5. Cover and add the mussels. Cook for 3 mins or until the mussels' shells open up. While they're cooking, gently shake the pan two or three times.
6. All the shells should be fully open at this point. Discard any mussels that are still unopened using a slotted spoon. Pour the broth over the mussels that have been opened in a shallow serving dish. If desired, garnish with more fresh lemon slices.

Nutrition: Calories: 22 Fat: 7 g Carbs: 6 g Protein: 18 g

6.16 Orange and Garlic Shrimp

Prep Time: 20 mins

Cook Time: 10 mins

Servings: 2

Ingredients:

- 1 large orange
- 3 tbsp extra-virgin olive oil, divided
- 1 tbsp chopped fresh Rosemary
- 1 tbsp chopped fresh thyme
- 3 garlic cloves, minced (about 1½ tsp)
- 1/4 tsp freshly ground black pepper
- 1/4 tsp kosher or sea salt
- 1½ pounds fresh raw shrimp, shells, and tails removed

Directions:

1. Using a citrus grater, zest the whole orange. Combine the orange zest, 2 tbsp oil, Rosemary, thyme, garlic, pepper, and salt in a large zip-top plastic bag.

2. Add the shrimp, zip the bag, and gently massage the shrimp until all the spices are evenly distributed and the shrimp is thoroughly coated. Remove from the equation.
3. Over medium heat, heat a grill, grill pan, or big skillet. The remaining 1 tbsp of oil may be brushed on or swirled in.
4. Cook for 4 to 6 mins, or until the shrimp become pink and white, turning halfway through if cooking on the grill or tossing every min if cooking in a pan. In a large serving dish, place the shrimp.
5. Add the remaining shrimp to the dish and repeat with the remaining shrimp.
6. Peel the orange and chop the flesh into bite-size pieces while the shrimp boil. Toss in with the cooked shrimp in a serving dish. Serve right now, or chill and serve later.

Nutrition: Calories: 190 Fat: 8 g Protein: 24 g Carbs: 9 g

6.17 Roasted Shrimp-Gnocchi Bake

Prep Time: 10 mins

Cook Time: 20 mins

Servings: 2

Ingredients:

- 1 cup chopped fresh tomato
- 2 tbsp extra-virgin olive oil
- 2 garlic cloves, minced
- ½ tsp freshly ground black pepper
- ¼ tsp crushed red pepper
- 1 (12-oz) jar roasted red peppers
- 1-pound fresh raw shrimp, shells and tails removed
- 1-pound frozen gnocchi (not thawed)
- ½ cup cubed feta cheese
- 1/3 cup fresh torn basil leaves

Directions:

1. Preheat the oven to 425 degrees Fahrenheit. Combine the tomatoes, oil, garlic, black pepper, and crushed red pepper in a baking dish. Roast for 10 mins in the oven.
2. Combine the roasted peppers and shrimp in a mixing bowl. Cook for a further 10 mins, or until the shrimp are pink and white.
3. Cook the gnocchi on the stovetop according to the package directions while the shrimp cooks.
4. Drain and keep heat in a colander. Take the dish out of the oven. Serve with the cooked gnocchi, feta, and basil.

Nutrition: Calories: 227 Fat: 7 g Carbs: 25 g Protein: 20 g

6.18 Spicy Shrimp Puttanesca

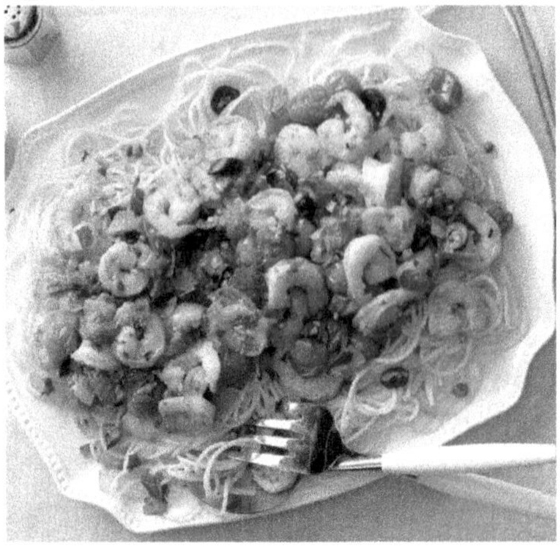

Prep Time: 5 mins

Cook Time: 15 mins

Servings: 2

Ingredients:

- 2 tbsp extra-virgin olive oil
- 3 anchovy fillets, drained and chopped
- 3 minced garlic cloves
- ½ tsp red pepper, crushed
- 1 (14.5-oz) can low-sodium or no-salt-added diced tomatoes, undrained
- 1 (2.25-oz) can slice black olives, drained
- 2 tbsp capers
- 1 tbsp chopped fresh oregano
- 1-pound fresh raw shrimp, shells and tails removed

Directions:

1. Heat the oil in a large skillet over moderate flame. Combine the anchovies, garlic, & crushed red pepper in a mixing bowl.
2. Cook, turning regularly, and crush the anchovies with a wooden spoon until they have melted into the oil, about 3 mins.
3. Toss in the tomatoes, olives, capers, and oregano, along with their juices. Raise the heat to medium-high and bring the mixture to a gentle simmer.
4. Stir in the shrimp when the sauce is just bubbling. Reduce the heat to medium-low and cook the shrimp for 6 to 8 minutes, or until pink and white, periodically tossing.

Nutrition: Calories: 214 Fat: 10 g Protein: 26 g Carbs: 20 g

6.19 Baked Cod with Vegetables

Prep Time: 15 mins

Cook Time: 25 mins

Serving: 2

Ingredients:

- 1 pound (454 g) thick cod fillet, cut into 4 even portions
- ¼ tsp onion powder (optional)
- ¼ tsp paprika
- 3 tbsp extra-virgin olive oil
- 4 medium scallions
- ½ cup fresh chopped basil, divided
- 3 tbsp minced garlic (optional)
- 2 tsp salt
- 2 tsp freshly ground black pepper
- ¼ tsp dry marjoram (optional)
- 6 sun-dried tomato slices
- ½ cup dry white wine
- ½ cup crumbled feta cheese
- 1 (15-oz / 425-g) can oil-packed artichoke hearts, drained
- 1 lemon, sliced
- 1 cup pitted kalamata olives
- 1 tsp capers (optional)
- 4 small red potatoes, quartered

Direction:

1. Preheat the oven to 375 degrees Fahrenheit (190 degrees Celsius).
2. Paprika and onion powder are used to season the fish (if desired).
3. Sear the top side of the cod for about 1 min in an ovenproof skillet over medium heat, until golden. Remove from the equation.
4. In the same skillet, heat the olive oil over medium heat. Stir together the scallions, 14 cup basil, garlic (if using), salt, pepper, marjoram (if using), tomato slices, and white wine. Removes from heat after bringing to a boil.
5. Spread the sauce evenly on the bottom of the pan. Scatter the feta cheese on top of the fish and tomato basil sauce. Place the artichokes in the skillet and top with the lemon slices.
6. Add the olives, capers (if using), and the remaining 14 cups of basil and mix well. Remove the pan from the heat and place it in the preheated oven. 15–20 mins in the oven
7. Meanwhile, cover the quartered potatoes in aluminum foil or lay them on a baking pan. Preheat your oven to around 350°F and bake for 15 mins.
8. Allow 5 mins to cool before serving.

Nutrition: Calories: 116 g Fat: 60g Protein: 64g Carbs: 10 g

6.20 Slow Cooker Salmon in Foil

Prep Time: 5 mins

Cook Time: 2 hours

Serving: 2

Ingredients:

- 2 (6-oz / 170-g) wild salmon fillets
- 1 tbsp olive oil
- 2 cloves garlic, minced
- ½ tbsp lime juice
- 1 tsp finely chopped fresh parsley
- ¼ tsp black pepper

Direction:

1. Place the salmon fillets in the center of a piece of foil on a work surface.
2. Combine the olive oil, garlic, lime juice, parsley, and black pepper in a mixing bowl. Brush the fillets with the mixture. To construct a package, fold the foil over and crimp the edges.
3. Cook on High for 2 hours after placing the package in the slow cooker.
4. Serve immediately.

Nutrition: Calories: 446 Fat: 21g Protein: 65g Carbs: 13 g

6.21 Crispy Fish Tacos with Grapefruit Salsa

Prep Time: 15 Mins

Cook Time: 20 mins

Servings: 4

Ingredients:

- 1/4 cup of tapioca flour
- Half cup of cassava flour
- Paleo Tortillas
- 3/4 cup of sparkling water
- 1 1/2 lb. of cod
- 1 tsp of sea salt

Grapefruit Salsa

- 1 chopped avocado
- 3 tbsp of chopped white onion
- 2 diced grapefruits, without skin
- Sea salt, to taste
- 2 tbsp of chopped fresh cilantro
- 1 tbsp of Lime juice

Directions:

1. Cut the fish into 8 pieces and gently cover in tapioca.
2. Whisk together the water, salt, and cassava in a mixing bowl.
3. Add enough oil to a pan to cook the fish.
4. Coat the fish in batter and cook for 3–4 mins on one side in hot oil.
5. Place it on a paper towel to absorb the liquid.
6. In a mixing dish, combine all the salsa ingredients.
7. Serve fish and salsa in warmed/grilled tortillas.

Nutrition: Calories: 265 Fat: 12.1 g Carbs: 14.9 g Protein: 21 g

6.22 Garlic-Butter Salmon and Asparagus

Prep Time: 10 mins

Cook Time: 15 mins

Serving: 2

Ingredients:

- 2 (6-oz / 170-g) wild salmon fillets, skin on and patted dry
- Pink Himalayan salt
- Freshly ground black pepper, to taste
- 1 pound (454 g) fresh asparagus, ends snapped off
- 3 tbsp almond butter
- 2 garlic cloves, minced

Direction:

1. Preheat the oven to 400 degrees Fahrenheit (205 degrees Celsius). Aluminum foil should be used to line a baking pan.
2. Season the salmon fillets on both sides.
3. Place the salmon in the center of the baking sheet and surround it with asparagus.
4. In a small saucepan over medium heat, melt the almond butter.
5. Garlic, minced, cooked
6. Drizzle the fish and asparagus with the garlic-butter sauce.
7. Preheat your oven to around 350°F and bake for 12 mins. To create a lovely sear on the asparagus, turn the oven to broil towards the end of the cooking period for around 3 mins.
8. Allow 5 mins to cool before serving.

Nutrition: Calories: 435 Fat: 26g Protein: 42g Carbs: 18 g

6.23 Lemon Rosemary Roasted Branzino

Prep Time: 15 mins

Cook Time: 30 mins

Serving: 2

Ingredients:

- 4 tbsp extra-virgin olive oil, divided
- 2 (8-oz) Branzino fillets
- 1 garlic clove, minced
- 1 bunch scallions
- 10 to 12 small cherry tomatoes, halved
- 1 large carrot, cut into ¼-inch rounds
- ½ cup dry white wine
- 2 tbsp paprika
- 2 tsp kosher salt
- ½ tbsp ground chili pepper
- 2 rosemary sprigs or 1 tbsp dried rosemary
- 1 small lemon, thinly sliced
- ½ cup sliced pitted kalamata olives

Direction:

1. Heat a large ovenproof skillet over high heat for 2 mins or until hot. 1 tbsp. extra virgin olive oil, heated
2. Sear the Branzino fillets for 2 mins, skin-side up. Cook the fillets on the other side. Remove from the equation.
3. 2 tbsp olive oil, swirled around the pan to evenly coat it.
4. Sauté for 5 mins with the garlic, onions, tomatoes, and carrot.
5. Stir in the wine until all the ingredients are fully combined. Place the fish on top of the sauce with care.
6. Preheat the oven to 450 degrees Fahrenheit (235 degrees Celsius).
7. Season the fillets with paprika, salt, and chili pepper and brush with the remaining 1 tbsp olive oil. A rosemary sprig and lemon slices should be placed on each fillet. Arrange the olives on top of the fish and all over the pan. Roast the lemon slices for approximately 10 mins, or until they are caramelized. Serve immediately.

Nutrition: Calories: 724 Fat: 43g Protein: 57g Carbs: 20 g

6.24 Grilled Lemon Pesto Salmon

Prep Time: 5 mins

Cook Time: 10 mins

Serving: 2

Ingredients:

- 10 oz (283 g) wild salmon fillet

- 2 tbsp prepared pesto sauce
- 1 large fresh lemon, sliced
- Cooking spray

Direction:

1. Preheat your grill to medium-high. Using cooking spray, coat the grill grates.
2. Season the fish with salt and pepper. On top, spread the pesto sauce.
3. Place the salmon fillet on a bed of fresh lemon slices approximately the same size as the salmon fillet on the hot grill. Any remaining lemon slices should be placed on top of the salmon.
4. Cook the fish for 10 mins on the grill.
5. Serve immediately.

Nutrition: Calories: 316 Fat: 21g Protein: 29g Carbs: 14 g

6.25 Paleo Crumbed Fish

Prep Time: 15 Mins

Cook Time: 25 mins

Servings: 5

Ingredients:

- 2 egg whites, whisked
- 12-14 oz of white fish fillets
- 2.8 oz of almond meal
- Salt, pepper, mixed dried herbs to taste
- Chopped walnuts, as needed

Directions:

1. Add almond meal to a mixing bowl.
2. Whisk the egg white in a separate dish.
3. Coat the fish with the almond meal before dipping it in the egg.
4. Walnuts, salt, pepper, and herbs are sprinkled on top.
5. Preheat oven to 375°f and bake for 8-10 mins, or until flaky.
6. Serve.

Nutrition: Calories: 331 Fat: 23 g Carbs: 3.9 g Protein: 25.8 g

6.26 Roasted Trout Stuffed with Veggies

Prep Time: 10 mins

Cook Time: 25 mins

Serving: 2

Ingredient:

- 2 (8-oz) whole trout fillets
- 1 tbsp extra-virgin olive oil
- ¼ tsp salt
- 1/8 tsp black pepper
- 1 small onion, thinly sliced
- ½ red bell pepper
- 1 poblano pepper
- 2 or 3 shiitake mushrooms, sliced
- 1 lemon, sliced

Direction:

1. Preheat the oven to 425°F (220°C). Using nonstick cooking spray, coat a baking sheet.
2. Olive oil should be applied to the interior and outside of the trout fillets. Salt & pepper to taste.
3. Combine the onion, bell pepper, poblano pepper, and mushrooms in a large mixing bowl. Fill the hollow of each fillet with half of this mixture. Inside each fillet, place 2 or 3 lemon slices on the mixture.
4. Place the fish side by side on the prepared baking sheet. Roast for 25 mins in a preheated oven.
5. Remove the dish from the oven and place it on a platter.

Nutrition: Calories: 453 Fat: 22g Protein: 49g Carbs: 5 g

6.27 Lemony Trout with Caramelized Shallots

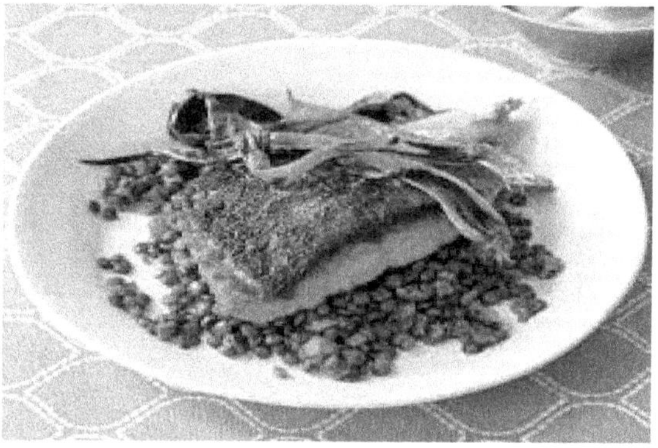

Prep Time: 10 mins

Cook Time: 20 mins

Serving: 2

Ingredients:

- Shallots:
- 1 tsp almond butter
- 2 shallots, thinly sliced
- Dash salt
- Trout:
- 1 tbsp almond butter
- 2 (4-oz / 113-g) trout fillets
- 3 tbsp capers
- ¼ cup freshly squeezed lemon juice
- ¼ tsp salt
- Dash freshly ground black pepper
- 1 lemon, thinly sliced

Direction:

1. Cook the butter, shallots, and salt in a skillet over medium heat for 20 minutes stirring every 5 minutes.
2. When it comes to trout,
3. Meanwhile, melt 1 tsp almond butter in a large pan over medium heat.
4. Cook the fish fillets for 3 mins on each side, or until flaky. Place the chicken on a plate and set it aside.
5. Stir in the capers, lemon juice, salt, and pepper in the same pan where the trout was cooked, then bring to a boil. In a separate bowl, whisk together the remaining 1 tbsp of almond butter. Using a spoon, drizzle the sauce over the fish.
6. Before serving, garnish the fish with lemon slices and caramelized shallots.

Nutrition: Calories: 344 Fat: 18g Protein: 21g Carbs: 9 g

6.28 Easy Tomato Tuna Melts

Prep Time: 5 mins

Cook Time: 4 mins

Serving: 2

Ingredients:

- 1 (5-oz) can chunk light tuna packed in water
- 2 tbsp plain Greek yogurt
- 2 tbsp finely chopped celery
- 1 tbsp finely chopped red onion
- 2 tsp freshly squeezed lemon juice
- 1 large tomato, cut into ¾-inch-thick rounds

Direction:

1. Preheat the broiler to its highest setting.
2. Combine the tuna, yogurt, celery, red onion, lemon juice, and cayenne pepper in a medium mixing bowl.
3. On a baking sheet, arrange the tomato circles. Toss some tuna salad on top of each one.
4. 3–4 mins under the broiler Allow 5 mins to cool before serving.

Nutrition: Calories: 244 Fat: 10g Protein: 30g Carbs: 7 g

6.29 Mackerel and Pinto Bean Salad

Prep Time: 10 mins

Cook Time: 10 mins

Serving: 2

Ingredients:

- 2 cups pinto beans
- 1 tbsp avocado oil
- 2 mackerel fillets
- 4 cups mixed salad greens
- 2 hard-boiled eggs, sliced
- 1 avocado, sliced
- 2 tbsp lemon juice
- 2 tbsp olive oil
- 1 tsp Dijon mustard
- Salt and black pepper, to taste

Direction:

1. Cook the pinto beans for 3 mins in a saucepan of boiling water. Drain the water and put it aside.
2. In a medium saucepan, melt the avocado oil. Cook the mackerel fillets for 4 mins on each side.
3. In two salad dishes, divide the greens. Add the mackerel, cut egg, and avocado slices on the top.
4. Drizzle over the salad with lemon juice, olive oil, mustard, salt, and pepper. Toss in the cooked pinto beans and serve immediately.

Nutrition: Calories: 737 Fat: 57g Protein: 34g Carbs: 16 g

6.30 Hazelnut Crusted Sea Bass

Prep Time: 10 mins

Cook Time: 15 mins

Serving: 2

Ingredients:

- 2 tbsp almond butter
- 2 sea bass fillets
- 1/3 cup roasted hazelnuts
- A pinch of cayenne pepper

Direction

1. Preheat the oven to 425 degrees Fahrenheit (220 degrees Celsius). The waxed paper should be used to line a baking dish.
2. Brush the fillets with almond butter.
3. In a food processor, combine hazelnuts and cayenne. Transfer the sea bass to the baking dish after coating it with the hazelnut mixture.
4. Preheat your oven to around 350°F and bake for 15 mins. Allow 5 mins to cool before serving.

Nutrition: Calories: 468 Fat: 31g Protein: 40g Carbs: 12 g

CHAPTER 7:

Meat & Poultry

7.1 BBQ Chicken & Vegetables Sheet Pan

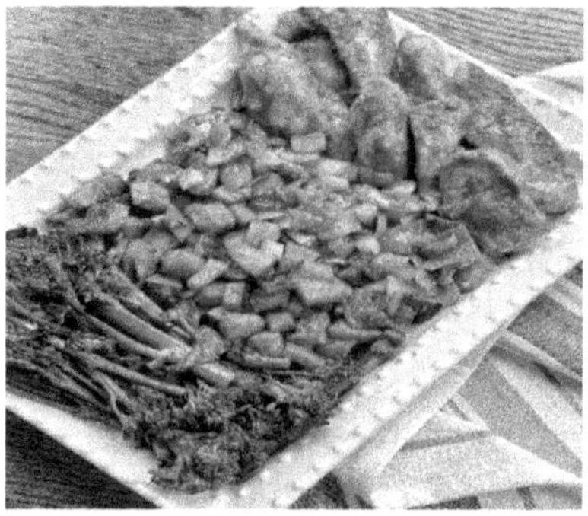

Prep Time: 45 Mins
Cook Time: 50 mins
Servings: 4

Ingredients:

- ⅓ cup of sugar-free BBQ sauce
- 1 tsp of salt
- 2 heads of broccoli, broken into florets
- 4 lemon slices
- Half tbsp of oil
- chicken thighs, boneless & skinless
- 2 cups of russet potatoes, diced
- Half tsp of thyme
- 1 tsp of garlic powder

Directions:

1. Mix the BBQ sauce into the chicken thighs well. Refrigerate for at least 30 mins.
2. Preheat your oven to around 350 degrees Fahrenheit.
3. Toss the potatoes with half of the garlic powder and salt (half) and the oil on one of the foil-lined baking sheets.
4. Spray the broccoli with oil, then place it on one side of the pan and stir with the remaining garlic and oil.
5. Place the chicken on one side of the same tray and brush with extra BBQ sauce.
6. Preheat oven to 400°F and bake for 40–50 mins.
7. Serve.

Nutrition: Calories: 378 Fat: 14 g Carbs: 6.9 g Protein: 32 g

7.2 Korean Beef Bowl

Prep Time: 15 Mins
Cook Time: 15 mins
Servings: 4

Ingredients:

- 2” of peeled fresh ginger, grated
- 1 tsp of onion powder
- 1 tbsp of sesame oil, toasted
- 2 pounds of ground beef
- 1 diced shallot
- 1 tsp of red pepper flakes
- 1 tsp of garlic powder
- Half cup of coconut aminos
- 2 cups of mixed greens
- 2 tbsp of fish sauce
- 4 cups of cauliflower rice

Directions:

1. Heat the oil in a pan over medium heat.
2. Break up the steak into tiny pieces and add it to the pan.
3. Add the shallots, ginger, onion, garlic powder, red pepper, and red pepper flakes. Cook for a further 8 mins.
4. Cook for 3 to 4 mins after adding the fish sauce and coconut aminos.
5. Beef with cauliflower rice and mixed greens is a delicious combination.

Nutrition: Calories: 392 Fat: 12 g Carbs: 7 g Protein: 38 g

7.3 Beef and Chili Mix

Prep Time: 15 mins
Cook Time: 16 Mins
Servings: 4

Ingredients:

- 2 green chili peppers
- 8 oz beef flank steak
- 1 tsp salt
- 2 tbsp olive oil
- 1 tsp apple cider vinegar

Directions:

1. In a skillet, pour the olive oil. Place the flank steak in the pan with the oil and cook for 3 mins on each side. The meat should next be seasoned with salt and apple cider vinegar.
2. Add the chili peppers to the skillet once they've been chopped. Cook the steak for another 10 mins. From time to time, stir it.

Nutrition: Calories: 166 Fat: 10.5g Carbs: 0.2g Protein: 17.2g

7.4 Creamy Tuscan Chicken

Prep Time: 15 Mins

Cook Time: 30 mins

Servings: 6

Ingredients:

- 1 tbsp of coconut oil
- 4 minced garlic cloves
- Sea salt & pepper
- 1/4 tsp of garlic powder
- 1 cup of chicken broth
- 1.5 lbs. of boneless & skinless chicken thighs
- 1/4 tsp of onion powder
- 1 chopped onion
- 1 tbsp of tapioca flour
- 1 1/2 cups of chopped baby spinach
- Half cup of coconut milk
- Half tbsp of ground mustard
- 1 1/2 tbsp of nutritional yeast
- Salt & pepper, to taste
- 1 tsp of Italian seasoning blend
- 2/3 cup of chopped sun-dried tomatoes

Directions:

1. Onion powder, salt, garlic, and pepper are used to season the chicken.
2. Heat the oil in a pan over medium heat. Cook for 5 to 7 mins on one side, then transfer to a platter.
3. Simmer until onions are soft, add garlic, and cook for 45 seconds.
4. Add the tapioca, coconut milk, and broth to the pot. Whisk everything together well.
5. Combine the Italian seasoning, mustard, salt, pepper, and yeast in a mixing bowl. Cook until the sauce begins to thicken.
6. Return the chicken to the pan, along with the tomatoes and spinach, and heat until the spinach has wilted.
7. Cook for another 2 mins before serving.

Nutrition: Calories: 368 Fat: 25 g Carbs: 12 g Protein: 23 g

7.5 Mediterranean Lamb Bowl

Prep Time: 15 mins

Cook Time: 15 mins

Servings: 2

Ingredients:

- 2 tbsp extra-virgin olive oil
- ¼ cup diced yellow onion
- 1-pound ground lamb - 1 tsp dried mint
- 1 tsp dried parsley -½ tsp red pepper flakes
- ¼ tsp garlic powder - 1 cup cooked rice
- ½ tsp za'atar seasoning
- ½ cup halved cherry tomatoes
- 1 cucumber, peeled and diced
- 1 cup store-bought hummus or Garlic-Lemon Hummus
- 1 cup crumbled feta cheese
- 2 pita bread, warmed (optional)

Directions:

1. Heat the olive oil in a large sauté pan or skillet over medium heat and sauté the onion for approximately 2 mins, until aromatic.
2. Mix in the lamb well, breaking up the meat as it cooks. Add the mint, parsley, red pepper flakes, and garlic powder after the lamb is halfway cooked.
3. Combine the cooked rice and za'atar in a medium mixing basin, then distribute into individual serving dishes. Toss in the seasoned lamb, then add the tomatoes, cucumber, hummus, feta, and pita to the bowls (if using).

Nutrition: Calories: 725 Protein: 62g Carbs: 62g Fat: 96g

7.6 Lamb Burger

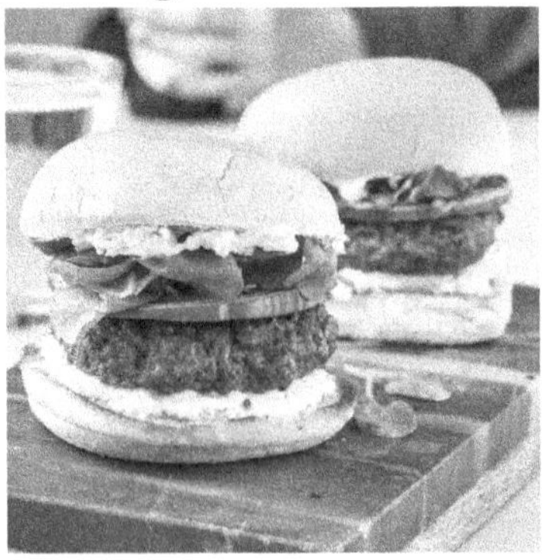

Prep Time: 15 mins

Cook Time: 15 mins

Servings: 4

Ingredients:

- 1-pound ground lamb

- ½ small red onion, grated
- 1 tbsp dried parsley
- 1 tsp dried oregano
- 1 tsp ground cumin
- 1 tsp garlic powder
- ½ tsp dried mint
- ¼ tsp paprika
- ¼ tsp kosher salt
- 1/8 tsp freshly ground black pepper
- Extra-virgin olive oil for panfrying
- 4 pita bread, for serving (optional)
- Tzatziki Sauce, for serving (optional)
- Pickled Onions, for serving (optional)

Directions:

1. Combine the lamb, parsley, oregano, cumin, garlic powder, mint, paprika, salt, and pepper in a mixing bowl. Make 4 tiny balls out of the meat and shape them into smooth discs.
2. Heat a sprinkle of olive oil in a large sauté pan or skillet over medium heat, coat a grill with oil, and set it on medium.
3. Cook for 4 to 5 mins on each side, or until the patties are cooked through, and the juices run clear. Tzatziki sauce and pickled onions are served on top of lamb patties in pitas (if using).

Nutrition: Calories: 328 Protein: 19g Carbs: 2g Fat: 27g

7.7 Marinated Lamb Kebabs with Crunchy Yogurt Dressing

Prep Time: 15 mins

Cook Time: 15 mins

Servings: 4

Ingredients:

- ½ cup plain, unsweetened, full-fat Greek yogurt
- ¼ cup extra-virgin olive oil
- ¼ cup freshly squeezed lemon juice
- 1 tsp grated lemon zest
- 2 garlic cloves, minced
- 2 tbsp honey
- 2 tbsp balsamic vinegar
- 1½ tsp oregano, fresh, minced
- 1 tsp thyme, fresh, minced
- 1 bay leaf
- 1 tsp kosher salt
- ½ tsp freshly ground black pepper
- ½ tsp red pepper flakes
- 2 pounds' leg of lamb, trimmed, cleaned, and cut into 1-inch pieces
- 1 large red onion, diced large
- 1 recipe Crunchy Yogurt Dip
- Parsley, chopped, for garnish
- Lemon wedges, for garnish

Directions:

1. Combine the yogurt, olive oil, lemon juice and zest, garlic, honey, balsamic vinegar, oregano, thyme, bay leaf, salt, pepper, and red pepper flakes in a bowl or big resealable bag. Mix thoroughly.
2. Add the lamb chunks and marinate for 30 mins in the refrigerator. Preheat the oven to 375 degrees Fahrenheit. Using skewers, thread the lamb onto the skewers, alternating with red onion pieces as desired.
3. Place the skewers on a baking sheet and roast for 10 to 15 mins, turning halfway through to achieve uniform cooking.
4. Allow the skewers to rest for a few mins after plating. Serve with a dollop of yogurt dressing on top. Garnish with fresh chopped parsley and a lemon slice to serve.

Nutrition: Calories: 578 Protein: 56g Carbs: 20g Fat: 30g

7.8 Garlic Pork Tenderloin and Lemony Orzo

Prep Time: 15 mins

Cook Time: 20 mins

Servings: 6

Ingredients:

- 1-pound pork tenderloin
- ½ tsp Shawarma Spice Rub
- 1 tbsp salt
- ½ tsp coarsely ground black pepper
- ½ tsp garlic powder
- 6 tbsp extra-virgin olive oil
- 3 cups Lemony Orzo

Directions:

1. Preheat your oven to around 350 degrees Fahrenheit. Drizzle the olive oil over the meat and season it with shawarma spice, salt, pepper, and garlic powder.
2. Place the pork on a baking sheet and bake for 20 mins, or until done to your liking. Allow the pork to rest for 10 mins after removing it from the oven. Assemble the meat and orzo on a platter and serve.

Nutrition: Calories: 579 Protein: 33g Carbs: 37g Fat: 34g

7.9 Roasted Pork with Apple-Dijon Sauce

Prep Time: 15 mins
Cook Time: 40 mins
Servings: 8

Ingredients:

- 1½ tbsp extra-virgin olive oil
- 1 (12-oz) pork tenderloin
- ¼ tsp kosher salt
- ¼ tsp freshly ground black pepper
- ¼ cup apple jelly
- ¼ cup apple juice
- 2 to 3 tbsp Dijon mustard
- ½ tbsp cornstarch
- ½ tbsp cream

Directions:

1. Preheat the oven to 325 degrees Fahrenheit. Heat the olive oil in a large sauté pan or skillet over medium heat.
2. Toss the pork into the pan and flip it to sear both sides with tongs. After the pork has been seared, season it with salt & pepper and place it on a small baking sheet.
3. Mix the apple jelly, juice, and mustard into the pan juices in the same skillet with the pork juices. Heat fully over low heat for 5 mins, stirring constantly. Pour the sauce over the meat.
4. Roast the pork for 15 to 17 mins, or 20 mins per pound, in the oven. Baste the pork with the apple-mustard sauce every 10 to 15 mins.
5. Remove the pork tenderloin from the oven and set it aside to rest for 15 mins. After that, slice it into 1-inch pieces.
6. Combine the cornstarch and cream in a small saucepan. Heat on a low setting. Stir in the pan juices for 2 mins or until they have thickened. Serve the pork with the sauce.

Nutrition: Calories: 146 Protein: 13g Carbs: 8g Fat: 7g

7.10 Moroccan Pot Roast

Prep Time: 15 mins
Cook Time: 50 mins
Servings: 4

Ingredients:

- 8 oz mushrooms, sliced
- 4 tbsp extra-virgin olive oil
- 3 small onions, cut into 2-inch pieces
- 2 tbsp paprika
- 1½ tbsp garam masala
- 2 tsp salt
- ¼ tsp ground white pepper
- 2 tbsp tomato paste
- 1 small eggplant, peeled and diced
- 1¼ cups low-sodium beef broth
- ½ cup halved apricots
- 1/3 cup golden raisins
- 3 pounds beef chuck roast
- 2 tbsp honey
- 1 tbsp dried mint
- 2 cups cooked brown rice

Directions:

1. Put the mushrooms and oil in an electric pressure cooker and set it to Sauté. After 5 mins, add the onions, paprika, garam masala, salt, and white pepper, and cook for another 5 mins. Continue to sauté after adding the tomato paste.
2. Add the eggplant and cook for another 5 mins, or until it has softened. Pour the broth in. Combine the apricots and raisins in a bowl. On each side, sear the meat for 2 mins. Close and seal the lid, then set the pressure cooker for 50 mins at high pressure.
3. Quickly remove the pressure when the cooking is finished. Take the cover with care, then remove the meat from the sauce and shred it. Stir honey and mint into the sauce as the meat is being removed.
4. Arrange 12 cups brown rice, 12 cup pot roast sauce, and 3 to 5 slices of pot roast on plates.

Nutrition: Calories: 829 Protein: 69g Carbs: 70g Fat: 34g

7.11 Shawarma Pork Tenderloin with Pitas

Prep Time: 15 mins
Cook Time: 35 mins
Servings: 8

Ingredients:

- For the shawarma spice rub:
- 1 tsp ground cumin
- 1 tsp ground coriander
- 1 tsp ground turmeric
- ¾ tsp sweet Spanish paprika
- ½ tsp ground cloves
- ¼ tsp salt
- ¼ tsp freshly ground black pepper
- 1/8 tsp ground cinnamon

- For the shawarma:
- 1½ pounds pork tenderloin
- 3 tbsp extra-virgin olive oil
- 1 tbsp garlic powder
- Salt
- Freshly ground black pepper
- 1½ tbsp Shawarma Spice Rub
- 4 pita pockets, halved, for serving
- 1 to 2 tomatoes, sliced, for serving
- ¼ cup Pickled Onions, for serving
- ¼ cup Pickled Turnips, for serving
- ¼ cup store-bought hummus or Garlic-Lemon Hummus

Directions:

1. For Make Shawarma, Combine the cumin, coriander, turmeric, paprika, cloves, salt, pepper, and cinnamon in a small bowl and put aside.
2. How to Make Shawarma:
3. Preheat the oven to 400 degrees Fahrenheit. Place the pork tenderloin on a platter and brush both sides with olive oil and garlic powder.
4. Season with salt and pepper and a good quantity of shawarma spices on each side of the tenderloin.
5. Place the pork tenderloin in the middle of a roasting pan and roast for 20 mins per pound or until it springs back when poked.
6. Cooking should be continued if there is still fluid beneath the skin. Check it every 5 to 7 mins until the desired softness is reached and the juices flow clear.
7. Allow the pork to rest for 10 mins after removing it from the oven. With pita pockets, tomatoes, Pickled Onions (if used), Pickled Turnips (if using), and hummus, serve the pork tenderloin shawarma.

Nutrition: Calories: 316 Protein: 29g Carbs: 17g Fat: 15g

7.12 Flank Steak with Artichokes

Prep Time: 15 mins

Cook Time: 60 mins

Servings: 4-6

Ingredients:

- 4 tbsp grapeseed oil, divided
- 2 pounds flank steak
- 1 (14-oz) artichoke hearts, drained and roughly chopped
- 1 onion, diced
- 8 garlic cloves, chopped
- 1 (32-oz) container low-sodium beef broth
- 1 (14.5-oz) can diced tomatoes, drained
- 1 cup tomato sauce
- 2 tbsp tomato paste
- 1 tsp dried oregano
- 1 tsp dried parsley
- 1 tsp dried basil
- ½ tsp ground cumin
- 3 bay leaves
- 2 to 3 cups cooked couscous (optional)

Directions:

1. Preheat the oven to 450 degrees Fahrenheit. 3 tbsp oil, heated over medium heat in an oven-safe sauté pan or skillet
2. On both sides, sear the steak for 2 mins each side. Preheat your oven to around 350°F and bake the steak for 30 mins, or until desired tenderness is achieved.
3. Meanwhile, add the remaining 1 tbsp oil, artichoke hearts, onion, and garlic in a large saucepan.
4. Combine the beef broth, tomatoes, tomato sauce, and tomato paste in a large mixing bowl. Combine oregano, parsley, basil, cumin, and bay leaves in a mixing bowl.
5. Cook the veggies for 30 mins, covered. If desired, remove the bay leaf and serve flank steak with 12 cups couscous per dish.

Nutrition: Calories: 577 Protein: 55g Carbs: 22g Fat: 28g

7.13 Easy Honey-Garlic Pork Chops

Prep Time: 15 mins

Cook Time: 25 mins

Servings: 4

Ingredients:

- 4 pork chops, boneless or bone-in
- ¼ tsp salt
- 1/8 tsp freshly ground black pepper
- 3 tbsp extra-virgin olive oil
- 5 tbsp low-sodium chicken broth, divided
- 6 garlic cloves, minced
- ¼ cup honey
- 2 tbsp apple cider vinegar

Directions:

1. Set aside the pork chops after seasoning them with salt and pepper.
2. Heat the oil in a large sauté pan or skillet over medium-high heat. Cook for 5 mins on each side, or until golden brown, before adding the pork chops.

3. Transfer the pork to a plate and decrease the skillet heat to medium-low after complete searing.
4. 3 tbsp chicken stock, added to the pan, will release the pieces and tastes stuck to the bottom of the pan.
5. Add the garlic to the pan once the stock has evaporated and simmered for 15 to 20 seconds, until fragrant.
6. Add the remaining 2 tbsp of broth, as well as the honey and vinegar. Return the heat to medium-high and cook for another 3 to 4 mins.
7. Stir the sauce occasionally until it has thickened somewhat. Return the pork chops to the pan, cover with sauce, and cook for another 2 mins. Serve.

Nutrition: Calories: 302 Protein: 22g Carbs: 19g Fat: 16g

7.14 Moussaka

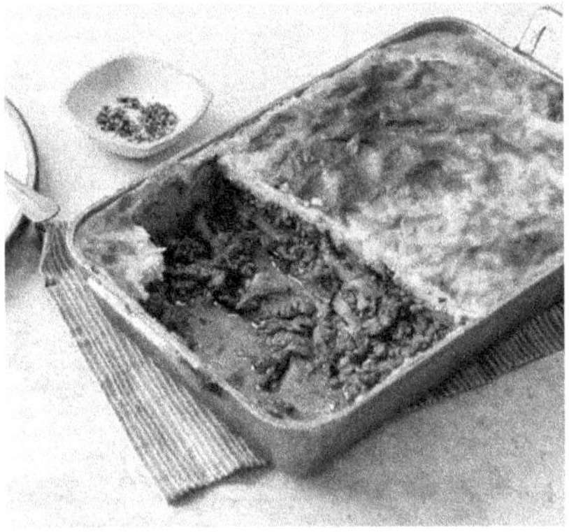

Prep Time: 15 mins

Cook Time: 40 mins

Servings: 6-8

Ingredients:

- For the eggplant:
- 2 pounds' eggplant, cut into ¼-inch-thick slices
- 1 tsp salt
- 2 to 3 tbsp extra-virgin olive oil
- For the filling:
- 1 tbsp extra-virgin olive oil
- 2 shallots, diced
- 1 tbsp dried, minced garlic
- 1-pound ground lamb
- 4 oz portobello mushrooms, diced
- 1 (14.5-oz) can crushed tomatoes, drained
- ¼ cup tomato paste
- 1 cup low-sodium beef broth
- 2 bay leaves
- 2 tsp dried oregano
- ¾ tsp salt
- 2½ cups store-bought béchamel sauce
- 1/3 cup panko breadcrumbs

Directions:

1. How to Cook Eggplant
2. Preheat the oven to 450 degrees Fahrenheit. Place the eggplant slices in a single layer on large baking pans lined with paper towels and season with salt.
3. Cover the eggplant slices with a second layer of paper towel. Continue this process until all the eggplant slices have been coated.
4. Allow 30 mins for the eggplant to sweat off any extra moisture. Make the beef sauce while this is going on.
5. Dry the eggplant with a paper towel. Place the eggplant slices on the baking sheets after drying them and brushing them with oil.
6. Bake for 15 to 20 mins, or until softened and gently browned. Remove the moussaka from the oven and let it cool slightly before assembling it.
7. Making the Filling
8. Heat the olive oil in a big, oven-safe sauté pan or skillet over high heat. Cook for 2 mins, or until the shallots and garlic soften.
9. Brown, the ground lamb, breaking it up as it cooks, with the garlic and onions. Cook, occasionally stirring, for 5 to 7 mins, or until the mushrooms have somewhat dehydrated.
10. Stir in the tomatoes and paste and the beef broth, bay leaves, oregano, and salt.
11. Reduce the heat to medium-low and cook for 15 mins, or until the sauce has thickened to your liking. Before assembling the dish, transfer the sauce to a separate bowl.
12. Reduce the oven temperature to 350 degrees Fahrenheit. Half of the eggplant slices should go in the bottom of the sauce saucepan. All the meat fillings should be placed on top of the pieces.
13. Pour the canned béchamel sauce over the remaining eggplant and place it on the meat filling. Breadcrumbs should be sprinkled on top.
14. Preheat oven to 350°F and bake for 30–40 mins, or until golden brown. Allow for a 10-min rest period before serving.

Nutrit

ion: Calories: 491 Protein: 23g Carbs: 30g Fat: 33g

7.15 Herbed Lamb Leg

Prep Time: 15 mins

Cook Time: 50 Mins

Servings: 4

Ingredients:

- 1 1/2-pound lamb leg, trimmed, meat only
- 1 tbsp Provance herbs
- 1 tsp salt
- 1 tbsp olive oil

Directions:

1. Season the meat with salt and Provance herbs. After that, brush it with olive oil and cover it in foil.
2. Preheat the oven to 360°F and bake the meat for 50 mins. Then toss out the foil and refrigerate the lamb meat for a few mins. Cut it up.

Nutrition: Calories: 336 Fat: 14.9g Carbs: 0 g Protein: 47.9g

7.16 Baked Pork Chops

Prep Time: 15 mins

Cook Time: 30 Mins

Servings: 4

Ingredients:

- 4 pork loin chops, boneless
- A pinch of salt and black pepper
- 1 tbsp sweet paprika
- 2 tbsp Dijon mustard
- Cooking spray

Directions:

1. Rub the pork chops with salt, pepper, paprika, and mustard in a mixing bowl.
2. Spray a baking sheet with cooking spray, place the pork chops on it, cover with tin foil, and bake for 30 mins at 400 degrees F.
3. Serve the pork chops with a side salad on individual plates.

Nutrition: Calories: 167 Fat: 5g Carbs: 2g Protein: 25g

7.17 Coconut Pork Steaks

Prep Time: 15 mins

Cook Time: 10 Mins

Servings: 4

Ingredients:

- 4 pork steaks (3.5 oz each steak)
- 1 tbsp ground turmeric
- 1 tsp salt
- 1 tbsp coconut oil
- 1 tsp apple cider vinegar

Directions:

1. Ground turmeric, salt, and apple cider vinegar are rubbed into the pork steaks. In a skillet, melt the coconut oil and add the pork steaks.
2. Cook the pork steaks for 5 mins on each side in the oven. Serve.

Nutrition: Calories: 366 Fat: 28.6g Carbs: 2.1g Protein: 25.1g

7.18 Sweet & Spicy Chicken Fingers

Prep Time: 15 Mins

Cook Time: 35 mins

Servings: 6

Ingredients:

- Half tsp of sea salt
- Half cup of honey
- ¼ tsp of black pepper
- 1 1/2 cups of almond flour
- Half tsp of garlic powder
- 1/4 cup of tapioca
- 1 lb. of chicken tenders
- 2 eggs
- ⅓ cup of hot sauce

Directions:

1. Preheat the oven to 425 degrees Fahrenheit.
2. Combine flour, salt, and pepper in a mixing basin.
3. Mix the eggs and 1 tsp of water in a separate dish.
4. Coat the chicken with tapioca starch, eggs, and a flour mixture. Place the breaded chicken tenders on a baking sheet lined with parchment paper.
5. Preheat oven to 350°F and bake for 25 mins. Add garlic powder, honey, and spicy sauce to a pan and stir over high heat.
6. Toss the chicken tenders in the sauce and bake for an additional 2 to 5 mins.
7. Serve with a side of sauce.

Nutrition: Calories: 287 Fat: 13.7 g Carbs: 11 g Protein: 27 g

7.19 Classic Chicken Cooking with Tomatoes & Tapenade

Prep Time: 25 mins

Cook Time: 25 mins

Servings: 2

Ingredients:

- 4-5 oz. Chicken breasts, boneless and skinless

- ¼-tsp salt (divided)
- 3-tbsp fresh basil leaves, chopped (divided)
- 1-tbsp olive oil
- 1½-cups of halved cherry tomatoes
- ¼-cup olive tapenade

Directions:

1. Arrange the chicken on a piece of waxed paper or glassine. Half of the salt and a third of the basil should be equally distributed over the chicken.
2. Flip the chicken pieces over with a little press. Add another third of the basil and the remaining salt. Another piece of waxed paper should be placed over the seasoned chicken.
3. Pound the chicken to a half-inch thickness using a meat mallet or rolling pin.
4. Heat some olive oil in a skillet over medium heat. Add the chicken breasts that have been pounded.
5. Cook for 6 mins on each side, or until the chicken is golden brown and no longer pink in the center. Place the browned chicken breasts on a plate and keep them warm by covering them.
6. Add the olive tapenade and tomatoes to the same skillet. Cook for another 3 mins, or until the tomatoes are just starting to soften.
7. Pour the tomato-tapenade mixture over the cooked chicken breasts and sprinkle with the remaining basil before serving.

Nutrition: Calories: 190 Fat: 7g Carbs: 6g Protein: 26g

7.20 Grilled Grapes & Chicken Chunks

Prep Time: 4 to 24 hours

Cook Time: 6 mins

Servings: 2

Ingredients:

- 2-cloves garlic, minced
- ¼-cup extra-virgin olive oil
- 1-tbsp rosemary, minced
- 1-tbsp oregano, minced
- 1-tsp lemon zest
- ½-tsp red chili flakes, crushed
- 1-lb. Chicken breast, boneless and skinless
- 1¾-cups green grapes, seedless and rinsed
- ½-tsp salt
- 1-tbsp lemon juice
- 2-tbsp extra-virgin olive oil

Directions:

1. In a small mixing bowl, combine and mix all the marinade ingredients. In a large mixing bowl, blend all ingredients until completely incorporated. Remove from the equation.
2. Using a 34-inch cube cutter, cut the chicken breast into 34-inch cubes. Thread the chicken and grapes alternately onto 12 skewers. To marinate the skewers, place them in a large baking dish.
3. Pour the marinade over the skewers, making sure they are well covered. Marinate for four to twenty-four hours.
4. Remove the skewers from the marinade and allow any leftover oil to drop off. Season with salt and pepper.
5. 3 mins on each side until the chicken and grape skewers are cooked through.
6. Place the skewers on a serving plate and sprinkle with lemon juice and olive oil before serving.

Nutrition: Calories: 230 Fat: 20g Carbs: 14g Protein: 1g

7.21 Turkish Turkey Mini Meatloaves

Prep Time: 15 mins

Cook Time: 20 mins

Servings: 2

Ingredients:

- 1-lb. Ground turkey breast
- 1-pc egg
- ¼-cup whole-wheat breadcrumbs, crushed
- ¼-cup feta cheese, plus more for topping
- ¼-cup Kalamata olives halved
- ¼-cup fresh parsley, chopped
- ¼-cup red onion, minced
- ¼-cup + 2-tbsp hummus (refer to Homemade Hummus recipe)
- 2-cloves garlic, minced
- ½-tsp dried basil
- ¼- tsp. Dried oregano
- Salt & pepper
- ½-pc small cucumber, peeled, seeded, and chopped
- 1-pc large tomato, chopped
- 3-tbsp fresh basil, chopped
- ½-lemon, juice
- 1-tsp extra-virgin olive oil
- Salt & pepper

Directions:

1. Preheat the oven to 425 degrees Fahrenheit.
2. Spray a 5"x9" baking sheet with non-stick greasing and line it with foil. Remove from the equation.
3. In a large mixing basin, combine and mix all turkey meatloaf ingredients except the 14-cup hummus. In a large mixing bowl, blend all ingredients until completely incorporated.
4. Divide the mixture into four equal parts. Make loaves out of the servings. On each meatloaf, spread a spoonful of the remaining hummus. Place the loaves on a baking sheet that has been buttered.
5. Bake for 20 mins, or until the centers of the loaves are no longer pink. (Use a meat thermometer to ensure the meatloaf is cooked through and the temperature hits 165 degrees.)
6. In a small mixing bowl, combine and mix all topping ingredients. In a large mixing bowl, blend all ingredients until completely incorporated.
7. Spoon the topping over the cooked meatloaves to serve.

Nutrition: Calories: 130 Fat: 7g Carbs: 14g Protein: 6g

7.22 Charred Chicken Souvlaki Skewers

Prep Time: min 8 hours

Cook Time: 15 mins

Servings: 2

Ingredients:

- ½-cup olive oil
- ½-cup fresh squeezed lemon juice
- 1-tbsp red wine vinegar
- 1-tbsp finely minced garlic (or garlic puree from a jar)
- 1-tbsp dried Greek oregano
- 1-tsp dried thyme
- 6-pcs chicken breasts, boneless, skinless, with trimmed off tendons and Fat
- Fresh cucumber and cherry tomatoes for garnish

Directions:

1. In a small mixing bowl, combine and mix all the marinade ingredients. In a large mixing bowl, blend all ingredients until completely incorporated.
2. Each chicken breast should be sliced crosswise into six 1-inch slices.
3. Place the chicken strips in a big plastic container with a tight-fitting cover.
4. Fill the plastic container halfway with marinade and close the top. Shake the container gently and flip it over to ensure that the marinade is equally distributed throughout the meat. Refrigerate the sealed plastic jar for 8 hours or longer to marinate.
5. Apply nonstick oil to the grill's surfaces. Preheat the grill, whether charcoal or gas, to medium-high heat.
6. Remove the chicken from the pan and set it aside to cool to room temperature. Drain the chicken and thread the skewers with it. (For each skewer, thread six pieces of chicken and fold each piece over so it does not spin around the skewer.)

Nutrition: Calories: 360 Fat: 26g Carbs: 3g Protein: 30g

7.23 Lemon Caper Chicken

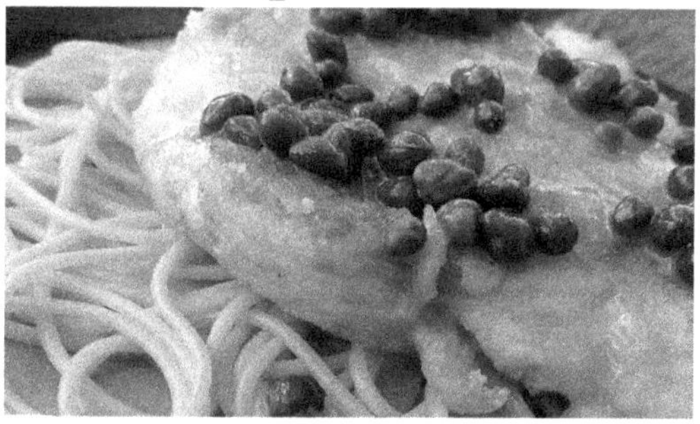

Prep Time: 10 mins

Cook Time: 15 mins

Servings: 2

Ingredients:

- 2 tbsp virgin olive oil
- 2 chicken breasts (boneless, skinless, cut in half, pound to ¾ an inch thick)
- ¼ cup capers
- 2 lemons (wedges)
- 1 tsp oregano
- 1 tsp basil
- ½ tsp black pepper

Directions:

1. Place a big skillet on the stovetop and pour in the olive oil. Set the temperature to medium and wait for it to warm up.
2. Season each chicken breast side with oregano, basil, and black pepper while the oil heats up.
3. Place your chicken breasts in a heated pan and cook for five mins on each side.

4. Remove the chicken from the pan and place it on a dinner dish. Serve with a couple of lemon wedges and capers on top.

Nutrition: Calories: 182 Carbs: 3.4 g Protein: 26.6 g Fat: 8.2 g

7.24 Herb Roasted Chicken

Prep Time: 20 mins

Cook Time: 1 hour

Servings: 2

Ingredients:

1 tbsp virgin olive oil

- 1 whole chicken
- 2 rosemary springs
- 3 garlic cloves (peeled)
- 1 lemon (cut in half)
- 1 tsp sea salt
- 1 tsp black pepper

Directions:

1. Preheat the oven to 450 degrees Fahrenheit.
2. Using paper towels, gently dry the entire chicken. Then add the olive oil and massage it's in. Remove one of the rosemary sprigs and distribute the leaves over the chicken. Season with a pinch of salt and black pepper. Place the entire remaining sprig of rosemary in the chicken's cavity. Then add the lemon halves and garlic cloves.
3. Place the chicken in a roasting pan and bake it for 30 mins. Allow 1 hour for the chicken to bake, then check for an internal temperature of at least 165 degrees F. Cover the chicken with foil and return it to the oven to continue cooking if it starts to brown too much.
4. Remove the chicken from the oven after it has reached the desired temperature. Allow for at least 20 mins of relaxation before carving.
5. Serve with roasted or steamed veggies on the side of your favorite salad.

Nutrition: Calories: 309 Carbs: 1.5 g Protein: 27.2 g Fat: 21.3 g

7.25 Italian Chicken Meatballs

Prep Time: 20 mins

Cook Time: 32 mins

Servings: 20

Ingredients:

- 3 tomatoes
- Kosher salt
- ½ cup of freshly chopped parsley
- 1 tsp of dry oregano
- Kosher salt
- ½ tsp of fresh thyme
- ¼ tsp of sweet paprika
- 1 red onion
- 1 lb. Of ground chicken
- ½ minced garlic cloves
- Black pepper
- 1 raw egg
- Extra virgin olive oil.

Directions:

1. Preheat the oven to 375 degrees Fahrenheit and grab a baking pan. Set aside after coating with extra virgin olive oil.
2. Combine the tomatoes, kosher salt, and thinly cut onions in a large mixing basin.
3. Sprinkle with half of your fresh thyme and a little extra virgin olive oil.
4. Transfer to your cooking and distribute with a spoon. Add ground chicken, egg, and oregano to the mixing bowl you just used.
5. Paprika, garlic, the other half of the thyme, chopped parsley, and black pepper are good additions.
6. Mix in a little quantity of extra virgin olive oil until the meatball mixture is well mixed. Form the mixture into 12-inch chicken meatballs and cut it to this size.
7. Obtain a second frying pan and place the meatballs in it. Combine the tomatoes and onions with the meatballs. Preheat your oven to around 350°F and bake for 30 mins.
8. Your meatballs should become golden brown; to make them more colorful, remove them from the oven and brush them with extra virgin olive oil before continuing to bake.
9. However, this isn't required. Your meatballs will be ready to eat in a few mins.
10. Your tomatoes are rapidly dwindling, which comes as no surprise.

Nutrition: Calories: 79 Carbs: 4.1g Protein: 7.8g Fat: 25g

CHAPTER 8:

Side Dishes

8.1 Pizzasallad Cabbage Slaw

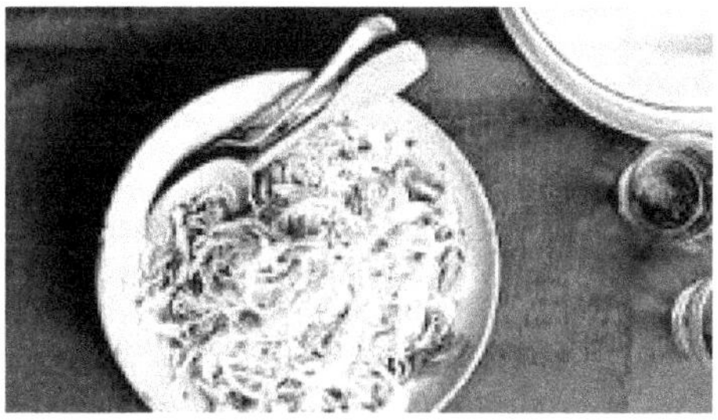

Prep Time: 20 Mins

Cook Time: 0 mins

Servings: 4

Ingredients:

- 2 tsp of sea salt - Half tsp of dried oregano
- Black pepper, to taste - 1 sliced red onion
- 1 pound of white cabbage
- 1 roasted sliced red bell pepper in oil
- 3 tbsp of olive oil - 1 tbsp of white wine vinegar - 1 tsp of sunflower seeds
- A pinch of red pepper flakes
- 1 tsp of poppy seeds

Directions:

1. Shred the cabbage finely in a food processor. Place it in a bowl and season with salt. Allow 20-30 mins of resting time before lightly squeezing to remove excess moisture and shake the salt.
2. Transfer to a mixing bowl and stir in the onion and red pepper.
3. Toss. Add the rest of the ingredients to a bowl, mix, and pour over the cabbage bowl.
4. Toss everything together and serve.

Nutrition: Calories 137 Fat: 11 g carbs: 10 g Protein: 2 g

8.2 Garlic Crispy Smashed Potatoes

Prep Time: 40 Mins

Cook Time: 45 mins

Servings: 6

Ingredients:

Potatoes

- 2 tbsp of Olive oil
- 12 Yukon small gold potatoes
- Sea salt, Fresh parsley & Black pepper, to taste

Cashew Cream

- 1 whole bulb of Garlic
- 2 tbsp of Fresh chives
- 3/4 cup of soaked Cashews
- 1 tbsp of Lemon juice

Directions:

1. Preheat the oven to 400 degrees Fahrenheit.
2. Remove any exterior papery coating of garlic and cut just 14" off the top. Wrap in foil after coating with olive oil.
3. Preheat the oven to 400°F and bake for 40 to 50 mins.
4. Add drained cashews to a food processor with a splash of boiling water and pulse until smooth. Combine the roasted, peeled garlic, chives, and the other ingredients in a mixing bowl. Pulse until the mixture is completely smooth.
5. Potatoes should be boiled for 8 to 10 mins. Drain and dry the potatoes before placing them on a baking pan to bake.
6. Lightly crush with a glass, then drizzle with oil and season with salt and pepper.
7. Bake for 30 mins, or until golden and crispy. Remove the tray from the oven and sprinkle with olive oil before broiling for 5 mins.
8. Garnish with a dollop of garlicky cashew cream.

Nutrition: Calories: 328 Fat: 12 g Carbs: 38 g Protein: 11 g

8.3 Tabbouleh Salad

Prep Time: 5mins

Cook Time: 12mins

Servings: 4

Ingredients:

- 1/4 cup olive oil
- 2 tbsp freshly squeezed lemon juice

- 2 garlic cloves, minced
- Pinch salt
- Pinch freshly ground black pepper
- 2 tomatoes, diced
- 1/2 cup chopped fresh parsley
- Cup dry bulgur wheat, cooked according to the package Directions

Directions:

1. Combine the olive oil, lemon juice, garlic, salt, and pepper in a mixing bowl. Toss in the tomatoes and parsley gently.
2. Toss in the bulgur to completely incorporate everything. Season to taste with salt and pepper if necessary.

Nutrition: Calories: 110 Fat: 12.1g, Carbs: 15.6g Protein: 7.6g

8.4 Caesar Salad

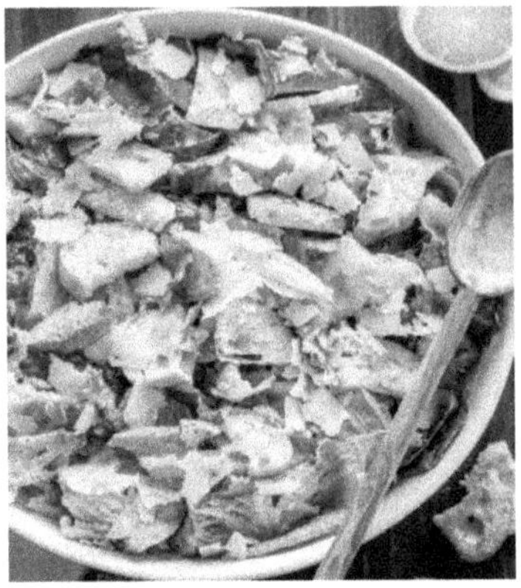

Prep Time: 10 mins

Cook Time: 5 mins

Servings: 4

Ingredients:

- 2 cups chopped romaine lettuce
- 2 tbsp Caesar Dressing
- 1 serving Herbed Croutons or store-bought croutons
- Vegan cheese, grated (optional)
- Make it a meal
- 1/2 cup canned chickpeas
- 2 additional tbsp Caesar Dressing

Directions:

1. To create the Caesar salad, follow these steps.
2. Combine the lettuce, dressing, croutons, and cheese in a mixing bowl (if using).
3. To turn it into a meal.

Nutrition: Calories: 120 Fat: 13.1g Carbs: 12.6g Protein: 7.6g

8.5 Greek Potato Salad

Prep Time: 10mins

Cook Time: 20mins

Servings: 3

Ingredients:

- 6 potatoes, scrubbed or peeled and chopped
- Salt
- 1/4 cup olive oil
- 2 tbsp apple cider vinegar
- 2 tbsp freshly squeezed lemon juice
- 1 tsp dried herbs
- 1/2 cucumber, chopped
- 1/4 red onion, diced
- 1/4 cup chopped pitted black olives
- Freshly ground black pepper

Directions:

1. Place the potatoes in a saucepan with enough water to cover them and a pinch of salt. Bring the water to a boil. Cook for 15 to 20 mins, or until the potatoes are tender. Drain the water and put it aside to cool. (Alternatively, toss the potatoes in a big microwave-safe dish with a little water.) Cover and microwave on high for 10 mins.)
2. Whisk together the olive oil, vinegar, lemon juice, and dry herbs in a large mixing basin. Combine the cucumber, red onion, and olives in a mixing bowl with the dressing.
3. Toss in the cooked, cooled potatoes to mix. Season to taste with salt and pepper if necessary.

Nutrition: Calories: 110 Fat: 17.1g Carbs: 19.6g Protein: 7.6g

8.6 Garlic Roasted Brussels Sprouts

Prep Time: 10 Mins

Cook Time: 20 mins

Servings: 4

Ingredients:

- 2 tbsp of minced garlic
- ¼ tsp of salt
- 2 lbs. Brussels sprouts, cut in half
- half tbsp of fresh chopped rosemary
- 1 tbsp of olive oil
- Half tsp of black pepper

Directions:

1. Preheat the oven to 400 degrees Fahrenheit.

2. Toss the Brussels sprouts with the other ingredients and lay them on a baking pan lined with parchment paper.
3. Bake for 15 minutes, then turn and continue baking for another 5-10 minutes.

Nutrition: Calories: 135 Fat: 4 g Carbs: 22 g Protein: 8 g

8.7 Shaved Brussels Sprout

Prep Time: 10 Mins

Cook Time: 10 mins

Servings: 4

Ingredients:

- 3/4 cup of chopped pecans
- Half tsp of salt
- 2 tbsp of balsamic vinegar
- 1/4 cup of hemp seeds
- cups of shaved Brussels sprouts
- 1 tbsp of olive oil
- 1 tsp of black pepper
- Half cup of dried cranberries
- Half tsp of rosemary

Directions:

1. 5 mins sautéing shaved Brussels sprouts in hot oil
2. Toss in the remaining ingredients, cook through and serve.

Nutrition: Calories: 109 Fat: 2 g Carbs: 1 g Protein: 3 g

8.8 Mashed Cauliflower

Prep Time: 15 mins

Cook Time: 15 mins

Servings: 5

Ingredients:

- 5 cups water
- 2 cups cauliflower florets
- 1 tbsp ghee
- Salt
- Freshly ground black pepper

Directions:

1. Bring 5 cups of water to a boil. Cook for 10 to 12 mins until the cauliflower florets are extremely soft. Return the cauliflower to the saucepan after draining it in a colander.
2. Mash the florets using a fork or a potato masher. Season with salt and pepper after adding the ghee. To blend, mash briefly.
3. Divide the mashed cauliflower evenly into two 24-oz single-serving meal prep containers. Refrigerate for up to 3 days before serving.
4. Reheat in the microwave in 30-second increments, stirring after each, until the mashed cauliflower reaches your preferred temperature.
5. Freeze: This is anything that can be frozen. Let it cool before transferring the mashed cauliflower to a quart-size resealable freezer bag. 1 month in the freezer. Refrigerate overnight to thaw.

Nutrition: Calories: 345 Fat: 67g Protein: 15g Carbs: 34g

8.9 Sheet Pan Rainbow Veggies

Prep Time: 15mins

Cook Time: 15mins

Servings: 6

Ingredients:

- 2 cups broccoli florets cut into large dice
- 2 cups whole button mushrooms
- 2 cups butternut squash, chopped small
- 1 zucchini, chopped small
- 1 yellow squash, chopped small
- 1 red bell pepper, chopped small
- 1 onion, chopped into 1-inch pieces
- 2 tbsp olive oil
- 2 tbsp balsamic vinegar
- 4 garlic cloves, minced
- 2 tbsp dried thyme - Salt
- Freshly ground black pepper

Directions:

1. Preheat the oven to 425 degrees Fahrenheit.
2. Toss the broccoli, mushrooms, butternut squash, zucchini, yellow squash, red bell pepper, onion, olive oil, vinegar, garlic, and thyme on the prepared sheet pan. Salt & pepper to taste. Arrange the veggies in a single layer on the baking sheet.
3. Roast until slightly browned, 12 to 15 mins.

Nutrition: Calories: 459 Fat: 34g Protein: 28g Carbs: 17g

8.10 Garlic-Lemon Roasted Broccoli

Prep Time: 5mins

Cook Time: 15mins

Servings: 4

Ingredients:

- 4 cups fresh broccoli florets

- 2 to 3 tbsp olive oil
- 2 garlic cloves, minced
- Juice of 1 lemon
- Salt
- Freshly ground black pepper

Directions:

1. Preheat the oven to 425 degrees Fahrenheit.
2. Toss the broccoli, olive oil, garlic, and lemon juice together on the prepared sheet pan. Salt & pepper to taste. On the sheet pan, arrange the broccoli in a single layer.
3. Bake for 12 to 15 minutes, shaking the pan every 5 minutes to ensure equal cooking.

Nutrition: Calories: 356 Fat: 17g Protein: 28g Carbs: 21g.

8.11 Savory Sweet Potatoes

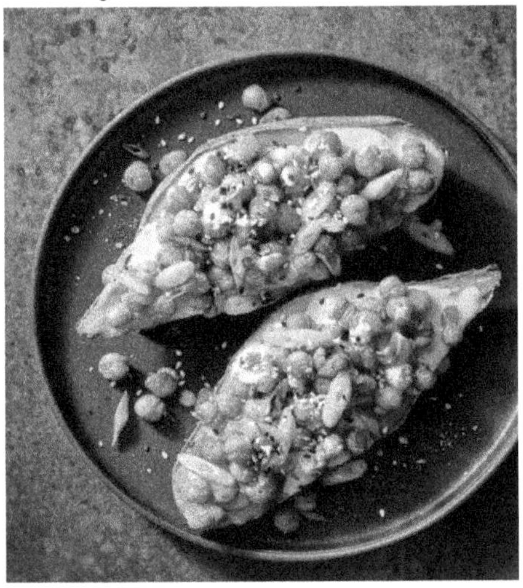

Prep Time: 10mins

Cook Time: 35mins

Servings: 4

Ingredients:

- 2 large, sweet potatoes cut into bite-size pieces
- 1 tbsp olive oil
- 1 tsp paprika
- 1 tsp dried thyme
- 1/2 tsp dried parsley
- 1/4 tsp salt

Directions:

1. Preheat the oven to 450 degrees Fahrenheit.
2. Toss the sweet potatoes with the olive oil on the prepared sheet pan to coat. Toss in the paprika, thyme, parsley, and salt until well combined. Make a single layer of sweet potatoes by rolling them out.
3. Preheat your oven to around 350°F and bake the sweet potatoes for 30–35 mins, or until they are soft.
4. Allow it cool before dividing into four 24-oz single-serving meal prep containers. Refrigerate for up to 4 days before serving.
5. Warm the sweet potatoes in the microwave for 60 seconds to reheat them.

Nutrition: Calories: 391 Fat: 34g Protein: 53g Carbs: 31g

8.12 Oven-Roasted Asparagus

Prep Time: 10mins

Cook Time: 8mins

Servings: 3

Ingredients:

- 8 oz' asparagus, rinsed, woody ends trimmed by 1 inch, dried
- 1/2 tsp salt
- 1/2 tsp freshly ground black pepper
- 3 garlic cloves, minced

Directions:

1. Preheat the oven to 425 degrees Fahrenheit.
2. Arrange the asparagus in a single layer on the sheet pan that has been prepped.
3. Combine the salt, pepper, and garlic in a small bowl.
4. Spray the asparagus lightly with cooking spray. The cheese mixture should be sprinkled on top. Mix the asparagus with the other ingredients with your hands and spread them out again in a uniform layer. Coat lightly with cooking spray once more.
5. Preheat oven to 350°F and bake for 8 mins.

Nutrition: Calories: 267 Fat: 56g Protein: 31g Carbs: 23

8.13 Simple Spaghetti Squash

Prep Time: 5mins

Cook Time: 50mins

Servings: 2

Ingredients:

- 1 spaghetti squash, rinsed, ends trimmed, halved lengthwise, seeds and pulp removed
- 2 tbsp olive oil or avocado oil
- Sea salt
- Freshly ground black pepper

Directions:

1. Preheat your oven to around 350 degrees Fahrenheit.
2. Drizzle olive oil over the squash halves cut side up, on a baking sheet or sheet pan. Salt & pepper to taste. Place the cut-side down squash halves on a cutting board.
3. Bake for 40 to 50 mins, or until a fork pierces the squash easily. Allow cooling after removing from the oven.

Nutrition: Calories: 191 Fat: 68g Protein: 42g Carbs: 23g

8.14 Fresh Black Bean Dip

Prep Time: 5 mins

Cook Time: 30 mins

Servings: 5

Ingredients:

- 1 small yellow onion, peeled and chopped
- 2 jalapeño peppers 1/4 cup red bell pepper
- 1 clove garlic, peeled and chopped
- 2 (15-oz) cans black beans, drained
- 3 tbsp water - 1 tsp ground cumin
- 2 tsp cocoa powder - 3 tbsp fresh lime juice
- 2 tbsp fresh chopped cilantro
- 4 cherry tomatoes, sliced

Directions:

1. Combine the onion, jalapeño, garlic, bell pepper, black beans, and water in a food processor bowl. Pulse three times, pushing down any contents that have risen to the top of the dish. Pulse in the cumin and cocoa powder until smooth.
2. Cook for 60 seconds in a medium microwave-safe container. Repeat the process. Remove from the microwave and set aside for 1 min to cool.
3. Lime juice and cilantro should be added at this point. Refrigerate for up to 5 days or freeze for 2 months if covered. To serve, heat in the microwave for 30 seconds until hot, then top with sliced cherry tomatoes.

Nutrition: Calories: 88 Fat: 0.3 g Protein: 5.5 g Carbs: 18.9 g

---

8.15 Easy Vegan Quest Dip

Prep Time: 5 mins

Cook Time: 15mins

Servings: 6

Ingredients:

- 1 package cream cheese vegan
- 1 can mild enchilada sauce green chili
- 3 tbsp yeast flakes
- 1 tsp garlic powder
- 1/2 tsp salt
- 1/4 tsp black pepper

Directions:

1. Microwave vegan cream cheese for approximately 20 seconds in a small microwave-safe bowl. Remove from the heat, mix, and continue until the sauce is smooth and easy to stir.
2. Over cream cheese, pour green chili enchilada sauce. To blend, stir everything together. Add the nutritional yeast flakes, garlic powder, salt, and pepper and stir to combine. Allow it cool for 5 mins before covering and storing in the refrigerator for up to 7 days.
3. Remove from the refrigerator and heat in the microwave for 30 seconds until cooked through.

Nutrition: Calories: 78 Fat: 0.3 g Protein: 2.5 g Carbs: 19.9 g

---

8.16 Vegan Seven-Layer Dip

Prep Time: 5 mins

Cook Time: 15mins

Servings: 10

Ingredients:

- 1 (12-oz) package vegan meat crumbles
- 1 tbsp olive oil
- 3 tbsp taco seasoning
- 1 can of black beans
- 1.1/2 cups mild chunky salsa, divided
- 2 cups vegan Cheddar shreds
- 1 cup vegan sour cream
- 1 cup guacamole
- 1 (2.25-oz) can black olives, chopped
- 1/2 cup chopped tomatoes
- 1/2 cup chopped green onion

Directions:

1. Brown vegan beef crumbles in olive oil in a large pan over medium heat for approximately 5 mins. Season with taco seasoning. Allow 5 mins for the mixture to cool to room temperature.
2. Combine the beans and 1/2 cup salsa in a blender or food processor. Blend for approximately 20 seconds, or until the beans are refried bean consistency.

3. Fill a large serving tray with beans that are approximately 11/2" deep. Top the beans with shredded cheese. On top of the cheese, scatter vegan meat crumbles. Spread sour cream on top of the vegan crumbles, then guacamole on top of the sour cream. Spread the remaining salsa equally over the guacamole. Olives should be sprinkled on top. Toss with tomatoes and green onions before serving. Refrigerate for up to 3 days if covered.

Nutrition: Calories: 58 Fat: 3.3 g Protein: 2.5 g Carbs: 17.9 g

8.17 Roasted Broccolini

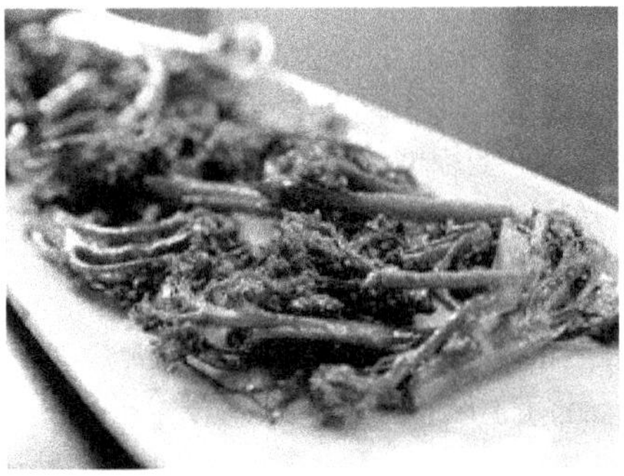

Prep Time: 10 Mins

Cook Time: 15 mins

Servings: 4

Ingredients:

- 2 tbsp of olive oil
- Salt & pepper, to taste
- 2 tsp of chopped garlic
- 2 bunches of broccolini
- Half lemon

Directions:

1. Preheat the oven to 425 degrees Fahrenheit.
2. Combine the broccolini, oil, salt, garlic, and pepper in a mixing bowl. Place on a baking sheet lined with parchment paper.
3. Preheat your oven to around 350°F and roast for 12 to 15 mins. Serve.

Nutrition: Calories: 102 Fat: 7 g Carbs: 7 g Protein: 3 g

8.18 Green Chili Hummus with Salsa

Prep Time: 5 mins

Cook Time: 15mins

Servings: 12

Ingredients:

- 1 (15-oz) chickpeas, rinsed and drained
- 2 tbsp tahini
- 2 tbsp nutritional yeast flakes
- 2 tsp garlic powder
- 1 (4-oz) can green chilies
- 1/2 cup fresh spinach
- 1 (8-oz) jar mild chunky salsa

Directions:

1. In a food processor, combine chickpeas, tahini, nutritional yeast flakes, garlic powder, green chilies, and spinach. 3 seconds of pulsing till grainy and crumbly
2. Set a colander on the counter and pour the salsa into it to drain the liquid.
3. In a food processor, add liquid 1 tbsp at a time and pulse until a spreadable consistency is achieved.
4. Fill a small serving dish halfway with hummus and top with strained salsa.
5. Refrigerate until ready to serve, covered (up to 4 days). It can also be frozen for up to a month.
6. Serve and have fun.

Nutrition: Calories: 169 Fat: 8.3 g Protein: 4.5 g Carbs: 20.9 g

8.19 Crostini with Pecan Basil Pesto

Prep Time: 5 mins

Cook Time: 15mins

Servings: 8

Ingredients:

- 1/3 cup pecans
- 1 cup fresh spinach
- 1/3 cup olive oil
- 1 tsp garlic powder
- 5 fresh basil leaves
- 1 baguette, sliced into 24 (1/2"-thick) slices

Directions:

1. Preheat oven to 350°F and roast pecans on an oiled baking sheet for 5 mins. Remove from the oven and set aside to cool for 2 mins.
2. In a food processor, combine cooled pecans, spinach, olive oil, vegan cheese, garlic powder, and basil leaves. To blend, pulse for 3 seconds.
3. Place bread pieces on a large ungreased baking sheet in a single layer. Place in the oven for 5 mins to toast. Remove from oven and let cool for 5 mins before transferring

to a medium covered container and storing in the refrigerator for up to 3 days.

4. Wrap bread in foil and cook for 5 mins in a toaster oven at 350°F, until toasted through. Serve with a dollop of Pecan Basil Pesto on top.

Nutrition: Calories: 65 Fat: 2.3 g Protein: 9.5 g Carbs: 14.9 g

---

8.20 Black-Eyed Pea Dip

Prep Time: 5 mins

Cook Time: 35mins

Servings: 6

Ingredients:

- 1 (15-oz) can black eye peas, drained
- 3 tbsp finely chopped peeled yellow onion
- 1/4 cup vegan sour cream
- 1/2 (8-oz) jar mild chunky salsa
- 1 cup vegan Cheddar shred.

Directions:

1. Place black-eyed peas in an ungreased 8" x 8" casserole dish and mash up most of the beans with a fork.
2. Combine the onions, sour cream, salsa, and 1/2 vegan Cheddar shreds in a mixing bowl. To blend, stir everything together. The leftover vegan Cheddar shreds should be sprinkled over the top of the mixture.
3. Bake for 25 mins, or until the top layer of cheese has melted. Allow 15 mins to cool after removing from the oven.
4. Refrigerate dip for up to 5 days in a big sealable jar. To serve, heat in the microwave for 30 seconds until well warm.

Nutrition: Calories: 105 Fat: 2.3 g Protein: 8 g Carbs: 18.9 g

---

8.21 Caramelized Onion Hummus

Prep Time: 5 mins

Cook Time: 35mins

Servings: 10

Ingredients:

- 1 small yellow onion
- 3 tbsp olive oil, divided
- 1 tsp agave nectar
- 1 (15-oz) chickpeas, rinsed and drained
- 1/4 cup pine nuts - tbsp lime juice
- 1/2 tsp dried basil
- 1 tbsp nutritional yeast flakes
- 1 clove garlic, peeled

Directions:

1. Place onions in a skillet over low heat. 1 tbsp olive oil drizzled on top. Cook for approximately 5 mins, or until the vegetables are soft. Then add the agave nectar and simmer for another 10 mins, or until it has caramelized. Remove the pan from the heat and put it aside.
2. Pulse chickpeas and pine nuts for 5 seconds in a food processor. 1/2 caramelized onions, remaining tbsp olive oil, lime juice, basil, nutritional yeast flakes, garlic, and remaining tbsp olive oil 3 seconds of pulsing till smooth Serve with the leftover caramelized onions on top. Refrigerate for up to 5 days in a medium-covered jar.

Nutrition: Calories: 79 Fat: 8.3 g Protein: 17.5 g Carbs: 18.9 g

---

8.22 Spicy Roasted Chickpeas

Prep Time: 5 mins

Cook Time: 35mins

Servings: 4

Ingredients:

- 1 can chickpeas - 11/2 tsp olive oil
- 1 tbsp Southwest Chipotle seasoning
- 1/2 tsp salt
- 1/8 tsp ground black pepper

Directions:

1. Preheat the oven to 400 degrees Fahrenheit.
2. In a medium mixing bowl, combine chickpeas and olive oil, stirring to coat each chickpea. Place chickpeas in the pan that has been prepared.
3. Preheat oven to 350°F and bake for 25 mins, or until chickpeas are crispy on the exterior. Remove from the oven and season with salt and pepper. Stir until everything is evenly covered. Season with salt and pepper, then refrigerate for up to 5 days in a small, covered container.

Nutrition: Calories: 167 Fat: 11g Protein: 15.5 g Carbs: 21 g

---

8.23 Southwestern Hummus

Prep Time: 5 mins

Cook Time: 15 mins

Servings: 10

Ingredients:

- 1 (15-oz) chickpeas, rinsed and drained

- 1/4 cup tahini
- 1/4 cup lime juice
- 1 cup mild chunky salsa
- 1 tbsp Southwest Chipotle seasoning

Directions:

1. Combine all ingredients in a food processor bowl and pulse for 3 seconds. Scrape down any ingredients on the bowl's side using a spatula. Pulse until the consistency is smooth once again.
2. Refrigerate for up to 5 days in a small, sealed container.

Nutrition: Calories: 234 Fat: 17 g Protein: 8.8 g Carbs: 23.5 g

8.24 Vegan Bacon Ricotta Crostini

Prep Time: 5 mins

Cook Time: 10 mins

Servings: 10

Ingredients:

- 1 baguette, cut into 24 slices
- 1 tbsp olive oil
- 1 clove garlic, peeled and chopped
- 8 slices vegan bacon
- 1 cup cashews
- 1/2 cup unsweetened almond milk
- 1 tbsp nutritional yeast flakes
- 1 tsp dried basil
- 1 tbsp mild miso paste
- 1/4 cup maple syrup

Directions:

1. Preheat the oven to 375 degrees Fahrenheit. Preheat your oven to around 350°F. Line a baking sheet with parchment paper.
2. Place slices on a prepared baking sheet and toast for 10 mins. Refrigerate for up to 5 days in a big sealable bag.
3. Preheat a medium skillet to medium-high heat. Add the garlic and olive oil. Remove from the equation.
4. Cook vegan bacon for 3 mins each side in the same skillet. Remove from skillet and leave aside for 5 mins to cool before breaking into pieces.
5. Combine soaked cashews, almond milk, nutritional yeast flakes, basil, and miso paste in a food processor bowl. 3 seconds of pulsing Repeat until the mixture is smooth and no big chunks of cashews remain.
6. Refrigerate for up to 5 days in a medium sealable container. To serve, spread one dollop of cashew ricotta on each toasted crostini, then divide vegan bacon bits and maple syrup on top. Toast for 5 mins in a toaster oven at 300°F until crispy.

Nutrition: Calories: 456 Fat: 11.9 g Protein: 17.9 g Carbs: 29.7 g

8.25 Vegan Beer Brats in a Blanket

Prep Time: 5 mins

Cook Time: 20mins

Servings: 10

Ingredients:

- 1/4 cup yellow mustard
- 1 tbsp agave nectar
- 1 (12-oz) bottle pale lager beer
- 4 vegan brats
- 8 dairy-free crescent rolls
- 1 cup dill and garlic sauerkraut
- 1 cup vegan mozzarella cheese
- 4 slices vegan bacon, halved

Directions:

1. Preheat your oven to around 350 degrees Fahrenheit.
2. In a small, lidded dish, combine mustard and agave nectar. Refrigerate for up to 7 days if covered.
3. In a medium saucepan, bring the beer to a boil over medium heat. Cook the brats after adding them to the pan. After each brat has been prepared, cut it in half. Remove from the equation.
4. Arrange dough pieces on a prepared baking sheet, evenly covering each with sauerkraut and vegan cheese.
5. Wrap a half-slice of vegan bacon around each brat. Place on a dough piece. Wrap each brat in dough firmly and squeeze to seal it. 15 mins in the oven
6. Allow 10 mins for cooling before transferring to a big, covered container and refrigerating for up to 5 days. Remove from refrigerator and cook in microwave for 30 seconds until well warm. Each roll should be slathered with mustard sauce.

Nutrition: Calories: 278 Fat: 5.9 g Protein: 20.1 g Carbs: 21g

8.26 Baked Jalapeño Poppers

Prep Time: 5 mins

Cook Time: 20mins

Servings: 10

Ingredients:

- 1/2 (8-oz) container dairy-free cream cheese, softened
- 1/2 (14.2-oz) container Diana Jalapeño Garlic Havarti Style Wedge, shredded
- 3/4 cup + 1 tbsp plain soy milk, divided
- 1/8 tsp garlic powder - 1/2 tsp salt
- 10 jalapeños, halved and seeded
- 2 tbsp ground flaxseed
- 1/2 cup all-purpose flour
- 1/2 cup breadcrumbs

Directions:

1. Preheat your oven to around 350 degrees Fahrenheit. Add vegan cream cheese, shredded vegan cheese, 1 tbsp soy milk, garlic powder, and salt in a medium mixing bowl. Stuff an equal quantity of cream cheese mixture into each half jalapeno.
2. Combine flaxseed and remaining soy milk in a separate medium bowl. Remove from the equation.
3. Fill a small dish with flour and another with breadcrumbs. Remove from the equation. A filled jalapeno should be floured first, then dipped in flaxseed mixture, then breadcrumbs. Place the breaded popper on the prepared pan and dip the remaining packed jalapenos in the same way.
4. Remove from the oven and set aside to cool. Refrigerate for up to 5 days in a big, sealed container. Heat for roughly 5 mins in a toaster oven at 350°F to serve.

Nutrition: Calories: 129 Fat: 873 g Protein: 12 g Carbs: 14g

8.27 Vegan Spinach Cheese Pinwheels

Prep Time: 15 mins

Cook Time: 20 mins

Servings: 10

Ingredients:

- 1/2 cup shredded vegan jack cheese
- 2 tbsp chopped green onion
- 1/4 tsp garlic powder - 1/2 tsp salt
- 1/4 cup all-purpose flour
- 1 Pepperidge Farm Puff Pastry Sheet
- 1 tbsp vegan butter, melted
- 1 tbsp plain soy milk
- 1 package frozen chopped spinach

Directions:

1. Combine vegan cheeses, green onions, garlic powder, and salt in a medium mixing bowl.
2. Sprinkle flour over a work surface to make it easier to work with. On a floured surface, lay out the pastry sheet. In a small dish, combine melted vegan butter and soy milk; brush over the pastry sheet, saving leftover mixture.
3. Spread the cheese mixture over the greased pastry sheet, then top with the drained spinach. Begin rolling the dough sheet from the side closest to you, wrapping the contents in as you go. Wrap the pastry roll in aluminum foil and place it in the freezer for 30 mins. Preheat the oven to 400 degrees Fahrenheit. Using veggie cooking spray, grease a baking sheet.
4. Cut the pastry roll into 1/2" slices using a sharp knife. Brush the slices with the remaining butter mixture and place them on the preheated pan.
5. Bake for 20 mins, or until the pinwheels are golden brown.
6. Remove from oven and set aside to cool for 5 mins before transferring to a big, airtight container. Keep refrigerated for up to five days. To serve, heat in a toaster oven at 350°F for 5 mins or until cooked through.

Nutrition: Calories: 143 Fat: 8 g Protein: 12g Carbs: 14g

8.28 Cheesy Kale Chips

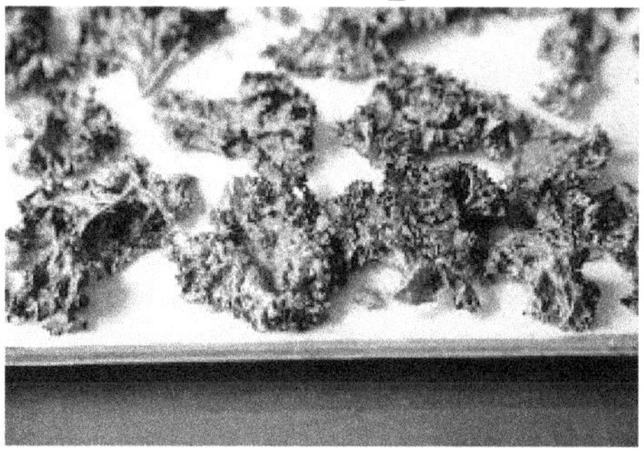

Prep Time: 10 Mins

Cook Time: 8-9 hours

Servings: 3-4

Ingredients:

- 1 cup of cashews

- 1/3 cup of water
- 1/4 tsp of bell pepper
- chili flake, to taste
- to 8 kale leaves, torn into big pieces without tough stems
- 2 tbsp of nutritional yeast
- 1 tsp of salt

Directions

1. Except for the kale, combine all ingredients in a food processor. Pulse until the mixture is completely smooth.
2. To get the correct consistency, add water.
3. Pour over the kale leaves and toss thoroughly to coat.
4. Place on an oven sheet and dehydrate for 8 to 9 hours at 140 degrees Fahrenheit with the oven door slightly ajar.
5. Serve.

Nutrition: Calories: 102 Fat: 3.4 g Carbs: 2 g Protein: 2 g

8.29 Carrot Hummus

Prep Time: 15 mins

Cook Time: 5 mins

Servings: 9

Ingredients:

- 1 (15-oz) chickpeas, rinsed and drained
- 1 cup roughly chopped peeled carrots
- 1 tbsp balsamic vinegar
- 2 tsp garlic powder
- 1/2 tsp ground cumin
- 1/2 tsp ground turmeric
- 1 tsp dried basil
- 1 tbsp tamari
- 4 tbsp water
- 2 tbsp olive oil

Directions:

1. Add all ingredients except the water and olive oil in a food processor and pulse until smooth. Remove the cover and whisk in the ingredients, adding 1 tbsp of water at a time until you get the required consistency.
2. Refrigerate for up to 7 days in a medium-covered jar. Drizzle olive oil over the hummus before serving.

Nutrition: Calories: 197 Fat: 20 g Protein: 16g Carbs: 11g

8.30 Vegan Cheesy Popcorn

Prep Time: 5 mins

Cook Time: 5mins

Servings: 2

Ingredients:

- 1/3 cup popcorn kernels
- 2 tsp nutritional yeast flakes
- 1 tsp paprika
- 1/2 tsp ground turmeric
- 1/8 tsp salt

Directions:

1. In a microwave popcorn popper, place popcorn kernels. Microwave for 3 mins with the lid on the container.
2. Combine the nutritional yeast flakes, paprika, and turmeric in a small bowl. To blend, stir everything together.
3. Remove the popcorn popper from the microwave using oven mitts, then gently remove the cover.
4. Remove the unpeopled kernels from the popcorn and pour them into a big sealable container. Using veggie cooking spray, liberally coat popcorn. Sprinkle the nutritional yeast mixture and salt on top, then evenly spread the spices throughout the popcorn using your hands or a spoon.

Nutrition: Calories: 210 Fat: 19 g Protein: 11g Carbs: 21 g

CHAPTER 9:

Rice, Bean, And Grain Recipes

9.1 Wild Rice, Celery, and Cauliflower Pilaf

Prep Time: 15 mins

Cook Time: 45 mins

Servings: 4

Ingredients:

- 1 tbsp olive oil, plus more for greasing the baking dish
- 1 cup wild rice
- 2 cups low-sodium chicken broth
- 1 sweet onion, chopped
- 2 stalks celery, chopped
- 1 tsp minced garlic
- 2 carrots, peeled, halved lengthwise, and sliced
- ½ cauliflower head, cut into small florets
- 1 tsp chopped fresh thyme
- Sea salt, to taste

Directions:

1. Preheat your oven to around 350 degrees Fahrenheit (180 degrees Celsius). Grease a baking sheet with olive oil and line it with parchment paper.
2. Pour the chicken stock over the wild rice in a saucepan. Bring the water to a boil. Reduce to low heat and continue to cook for another 30 mins, or until the rice is plump.
3. Meanwhile, heat the remaining olive oil over medium-high heat in an oven-safe pan until it shimmers.
4. In a large pan, sauté the onion, celery, and garlic for 3 mins, or until the onion is transparent.
5. Cook for 5 mins with the carrots and cauliflower in the skillet. Remove the pan from the heat and put it aside.
6. Combine the cooked rice and the veggies in a pan. Season with salt and thyme. Preheat your oven to around 350°F and bake the skillet for 15 mins, or until the veggies are tender. Serve right away.

Nutrition: Calories: 214 Fat: 3.9g Protein: 7.2g Carbs: 37.9g

9.2 Slow Cooked Turkey and Brown Rice

Prep Time: 15 mins

Cook Time: 3 hours & 10 mins

Servings: 6

Ingredients:

- 1 tbsp extra-virgin olive oil
- 1½ pounds (680 g) ground turkey
- 2 tbsp chopped fresh sage, divided
- 2 tbsp chopped fresh thyme, divided
- 1 tsp sea salt
- ½ tsp ground black pepper
- 2 cups brown rice
- 1 (14-oz / 397-g) can stewed tomatoes, with the juice
- ¼ cup pitted and sliced Kalamata olives
- 3 medium zucchinis, sliced thinly
- ¼ cup chopped fresh flat-leaf parsley
- 1 medium yellow onion, chopped
- 1 tbsp plus 1 tsp balsamic vinegar
- 2 cups low-sodium chicken stock
- 2 garlic cloves, minced

Directions:

1. Heat the olive oil over medium-high heat in a nonstick skillet until it shimmers. Sprinkle 1 tbsp sage, 1 tbsp thyme, salt, and ground black pepper over the ground turkey.
2. Cook for 10 mins, or until the turkey is gently browned. After that, add the other ingredients to the slow cooker. Stir everything together well.
3. Cover and simmer for 3 hours on high, or until the rice and veggies are cooked. Spread them out in a big serving basin.

Nutrition: Calories: 499 Fat: 16.4g Protein: 32.4g Carbs: 56.5g

9.3 Papaya, Jicama, and Peas Rice Bowl

Prep Time: 15 mins

Cook Time: 45 mins

Servings: 4

Ingredients:

- Sauce:
- Juice of ¼ lemon
- 2 tsp chopped fresh basil
- 1 tbsp raw honey
- 1 tbsp extra-virgin olive oil
- Sea salt, to taste
- Rice:
- 1½ cups wild rice
- 2 papayas, peeled, seeded, and diced
- 1 jicama, peeled and shredded
- 1 cup snow peas, julienned
- 2 cups shredded cabbage
- 1 scallion, white and green parts, chopped

Directions:

1. In a mixing dish, combine the sauce ingredients. Stir everything together well. Keep it aside until you're ready to utilize it. Fill a pot halfway with water, then add the wild rice. Bring the water to a boil.
2. Reduce the heat to low and cook the wild rice for 45 mins, or until it is soft and plump. Drain the pasta and place it in a big serving bowl.
3. Papayas, jicama, peas, cabbage, and scallion go on top of the rice. Before serving, pour the sauce over the top and stir well to combine.

Nutrition: Calories: 446 Fat: 7.9g Protein: 13.1g Carbs: 85.8g

9.4 Italian Baked Beans

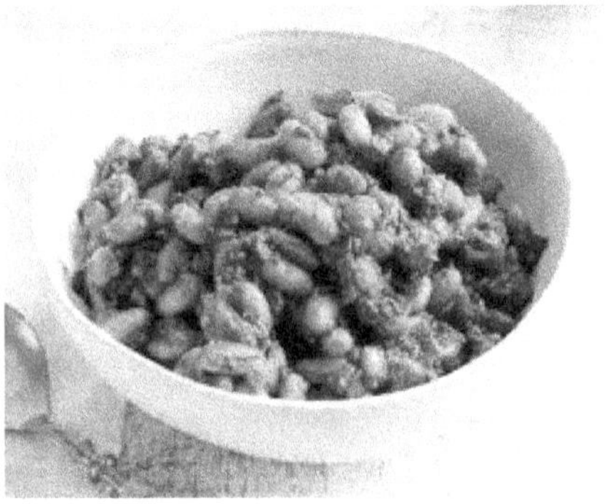

Prep Time: 5 mins

Cook Time: 15 mins

Servings: 6

Ingredients:

- 2 tsp extra-virgin olive oil
- ½ cup minced onion (about ¼ onion)
- 1 (12-oz) can low-sodium tomato paste
- ¼ cup red wine vinegar
- 2 tbsp honey
- ¼ tsp ground cinnamon
- ½ cup water
- 2 (15-oz) cans cannellini or great northern beans, undrained

Directions:

1. Heat the oil in a medium saucepan over medium heat. Cook, constantly stirring, for 5 mins after adding the onion.
2. Mix the tomato paste, vinegar, honey, cinnamon, and water until well combined. Reduce the heat to a low setting. In a strainer, drain and rinse one can of beans before adding to the pot.
3. Fill the pot halfway with the second can of beans (including the liquid). Allow for 10 mins of cooking time, stirring periodically, before serving.
4. Make fresh variants of the homemade ketchup to add variety to this dish. Try 14 tsp smoked paprika and 1 tbsp spicy sauce in place of the cinnamon. Serve.

Nutrition: Calories: 236 Fat: 3g Carbs: 42g Protein: 10g

9.5 Cannellini Bean Lettuce Wraps

Prep Time: 15 mins

Cook Time: 10 mins

Servings: 4

Ingredients:

- 1 tbsp extra-virgin olive oil
- ½ cup diced red onion (about ¼ onion)
- ¾ cup chopped fresh tomatoes (about 1 medium tomato)
- ¼ tsp freshly ground black pepper
- 1 (15-oz) cannellini or great northern beans, drained and rinsed
- ¼ cup finely chopped fresh curly parsley
- ½ cup Lemony Garlic Hummus or ½ cup prepared hummus
- 8 romaine lettuce leaves

Directions:

1. Heat the oil in a large skillet over medium heat. Cook, stirring periodically, for 3 mins after adding the onion.
2. Cook for 3 mins longer, stirring regularly, after adding the tomatoes and pepper. Cook, stirring periodically, for another 3 mins after adding the beans. Remove the pan from the heat and add the parsley.

3. Using 1 tbsp of hummus, coat each lettuce leaf. Distribute the heated bean mixture evenly over the middle of each leaf.
4. Fold one side of the lettuce leaf lengthwise over the filling, then fold the other side over to form a wrap and serve.

Nutrition: Calories: 211 Fat: 8g Carbs: 28g Protein: 10g

9.6 Israeli Eggplant, Chickpea, and Mint Sauté

Prep Time: 5 mins

Cook Time: 20 mins

Servings: 6

Ingredients:

- Nonstick cooking spray
- 1 medium globe eggplant (about 1 pound), stem removed
- 1 tbsp olive oil extra-virgin
- 2 tbsp lemon juice freshly squeezed
- 2 tbsp balsamic vinegar
- 1 tsp ground cumin
- 1/4 tsp kosher or sea salt
- 1 (15-oz) can chickpeas, drained and rinsed
- 1 cup sliced sweet onion (about 1/2 medium Walla Walla or Vidalia onion)
- 1/4 cup loosely packed chopped or torn mint leaves
- 1 tbsp sesame seeds, toasted if desired
- 1 garlic clove, finely minced (about 1/2 tsp)

Directions:

1. One oven rack should be placed approximately 4 inches below the broiler element. To preheat the broiler, put it to the maximum setting. Using nonstick cooking spray, coat a large, rimmed baking sheet.
2. Cut the eggplant lengthwise into four slabs on a cutting board (each piece should be approximately 12 to 1/8-inch thick). Place the eggplant slabs on the baking sheet that has been prepared. Remove from the equation.
3. Whisk together the oil, lemon juice, vinegar, cumin, and salt in a small basin. 2 tbsp lemon dressing brushed or drizzled over both sides of the eggplant slabs. Keep the rest of the dressing aside.
4. Broil the eggplant for 4 mins directly under the heat source, then turn and broil for another 4 mins, or until golden brown.
5. Combine the chickpeas, onion, mint, sesame seeds, and garlic in a serving dish while the eggplant is broiling. Mix in the reserved dressing until all the ingredients are well combined.
6. When the eggplant is done, remove the slabs from the baking sheet with tongs and place them on a cooling rack to cool for 3 mins.
7. Place the eggplant on a cutting board and slice each slab crosswise into 12-inch strips after it has cooled somewhat.
8. Combine the eggplant with the onion mixture in a serving basin. Serve warm or at room temperature after gently tossing everything together.

Nutrition: Calories: 159 Fat: 4g Carbs: 26g Protein: 6g

9.7 Mediterranean Lentils and Rice

Prep Time: 5 mins

Cook Time: 25 mins

Servings: 4

Ingredients:

- 2 1/4 cups low-sodium or no-salt-added vegetable broth
- 1/2 cup uncooked brown or green lentils
- 1/2 cup uncooked instant brown rice
- 1/2 cup diced carrots (about 1 carrot)
- 1/2 cup diced celery (about 1 stalk)
- 1 (2.25-oz) can sliced olives, drained (about 1/2 cup)
- 1/4 cup diced red onion (about 1/8 onion)
- 1/4 cup chopped fresh curly-leaf parsley
- 1 1/2 tbsp extra-virgin olive oil
- 1 tbsp freshly squeezed lemon juice (from about 1/2 small lemon)
- 1 garlic clove, minced (about 1/2 tsp)
- 1/4 tsp kosher or sea salt
- 1/4 tsp freshly ground black pepper

Directions:

1. Bring the broth and lentils to a boil in a medium saucepan over high heat, then cover and reduce to medium-low heat. Cook for a further 8 mins.
2. Raise the heat to medium and add the rice, stirring constantly. Cover the saucepan and simmer for 15 mins, or until all the liquid has been absorbed. Remove the saucepan from the heat and cover it aside for 1 min before stirring.
3. In a large serving dish, combine the carrots, celery, olives, onion, and parsley while the lentils and rice are cooking.

4. Whisk the oil, lemon juice, garlic, salt, and pepper in a small bowl. Remove from the equation. Add the lentils and rice to the serving dish after cooking.
5. Mix everything after pouring the dressing over the top. Serve warm or cold or refrigerated for up to 7 days in an airtight container.

Nutrition: Calories: 230 Fat: 8g Carbs: 34g Protein: 8g

9.8 Brown Rice Pilaf with Golden Raisins

Prep Time: 5 mins

Cook Time: 15 mins

Servings: 6

Ingredients:

- 1 tbsp extra-virgin olive oil
- 1 cup chopped onion (about ½ medium onion)
- ½ cup shredded carrot (about 1 medium carrot) - 1 tsp ground cumin
- ½ tsp ground cinnamon
- 2 cups instant brown rice
- 1¾ cups 100% orange juice
- ¼ cup water
- 1 cup golden raisins
- ½ cup shelled pistachios
- Chopped fresh chives (optional)

Directions:

1. Heat the oil in a medium saucepan over medium-high heat. Cook, constantly stirring, for 5 mins after adding the onion.
2. Cook for 1 min, constantly stirring, after adding the carrot, cumin, and cinnamon. Combine the rice, orange juice, and water in a mixing bowl.
3. Bring to a boil, cover, and reduce to medium-low heat. Cook for 7 mins, or until the rice is tender and the liquid has evaporated. Serve with the raisins, pistachios, and chives if used.

Nutrition: Calories: 320 Fat: 7g Carbs: 61g Protein: 6g

9.9 Quinoa and Chickpea Vegetable Bowls

Prep Time: 15 mins

Cook Time: 15 mins

Servings: 4

Ingredients:

- 1 cup red dry quinoa, rinsed and drained
- 2 cups low-sodium vegetable soup
- 2 cups fresh spinach
- 2 cups finely shredded red cabbage
- 1 (15-oz / 425-g) can chickpeas, drained and rinsed
- 1 ripe avocado, thinly sliced
- 1 cup shredded carrots
- 1 red bell pepper, thinly sliced
- 4 tbsp Mango Sauce
- ½ cup fresh cilantro, chopped
- Mango Sauce:
- 1 mango, diced
- ¼ cup fresh lime juice
- ½ tsp ground turmeric
- 1 tsp finely minced fresh ginger
- ¼ tsp sea salt
- Pinch of ground red pepper
- 1 tsp pure maple syrup
- 2 tbsp extra-virgin olive oil

Directions:

1. In a saucepan, combine the quinoa and vegetable soup. Bring the water to a boil. Reduce the heat to a low setting. Cook, covered, for 15 mins or until vegetables are soft. With a fork, fluffy
2. In a food processor, mix the ingredients for the mango sauce. Pulse until the mixture is completely smooth.
3. Fill 4 serving bowls halfway with quinoa, spinach, and cabbage, then top with chickpeas, avocado, carrots, and bell pepper.
4. Spread the mango sauce on top and garnish with cilantro. Serve right away.

Nutrition: Calories: 366 Fat: 11.1g Protein: 15.5g Carbs: 55.6g

9.10 Ritzy Veggie Chili

Prep Time: 15 mins

Cook Time: 5 hours

Servings: 4

Ingredients:

- 1 (28-oz / 794-g) can chopped tomatoes, with the juice
- 1 (15-oz / 425-g) can black beans, drained and rinsed
- 1 (15-oz / 425-g) can redly beans, drained and rinsed
- 1 medium green bell pepper, chopped
- 1 yellow onion, chopped
- 1 tbsp onion powder
- 1 tsp paprika

- 1 tsp cayenne pepper
- 1 tsp garlic powder
- ½ tsp sea salt
- ½ tsp ground black pepper
- 1 tbsp olive oil
- 1 large Hass avocado, pitted, peeled, and chopped, for garnish

Directions:

1. In a slow cooker, combine all the ingredients except the avocado. Stir everything together well.
2. Place the cover on the slow cooker and simmer on high for 5 hours, or until the veggies are soft and the mixture has thickened.
3. In a large serving dish, pour the chili. Allow 30 mins to cool before spreading with diced avocado and serving.

Nutrition: Calories: 633 Fat: 16.3g Protein: 31.7g Carbs: 97.0g

9.11 Spicy Italian Bean Balls with Marinara

Prep Time: 15 mins

Cook Time: 45 mins

Servings: 2-4

Ingredients:

- Bean Balls:
- 1 tbsp extra-virgin olive oil
- ½ yellow onion, minced
- 1 tsp fennel seeds
- 2 tsp oregano dried
- ½ tsp pepper flakes crushed
- 1 tsp garlic powder
- 1 (15-oz / 425-g) can white beans (cannellini or navy), drained and rinsed
- ½ cup whole-grain breadcrumbs
- Sea salt and black pepper
- Marinara:
- 1 tbsp olive oil extra-virgin
- 3 minced garlic cloves
- Handful basil leaves
- 1 (28-oz / 794-g) can chopped tomatoes with juice reserved
- Sea salt, to taste

Directions:

1. Preheat your oven to around 350 degrees Fahrenheit (180 degrees Celsius). Using parchment paper, line a baking sheet. Heat the olive oil over moderate heat in a nonstick skillet until it shimmers.
2. Sauté for 5 mins, or unless the onion is transparent. Cook for 1 min, or until fragrant, adding fennel seeds, oregano, pepper flakes, and garlic powder.
3. Combine the sautéed mixture with the beans and breadcrumbs in a food processor. Season with salt and powdered black pepper, then pulse until the mixture is completely combined and holds together. Using a 2-oz (57-g) cookie scoop, form the dough into balls and place them on the baking sheet.
4. Bake for 30 mins or until gently browned in a preheated oven. Halfway through the cooking period, flip the balls.
5. Warm the olive oil in a saucepan over medium-high heat while baking the bean balls. Sauté for 2 mins, or until garlic and basil are aromatic.
6. Combine the tomatoes and juice in a mixing bowl. Bring the water to a boil. Reduce the heat to a low setting. Simmer for 15 mins with the cover on.

Nutrition: Calories: 351 Fat: 16.4g Protein: 11.5g Carbs: 42.9g

9.12 Baked Rolled Oat with Pears and Pecans

Prep Time: 15 mins

Cook Time: 30 mins

Servings: 6

Ingredients:

- 2 tbsp coconut oil, melted, plus more for greasing the pan
- 3 ripe pears, cored and diced
- 2 cups unsweetened almond milk
- 1 tbsp pure vanilla extract
- ¼ cup pure maple syrup
- 2 cups gluten-free rolled oats
- ½ cup raisins - ¾ cup chopped pecans
- ¼ tsp ground nutmeg
- 1 tsp ground cinnamon
- ½ tsp ground ginger
- ¼ tsp sea salt

Directions:

1. Preheat your oven to around 350 degrees Fahrenheit (180 degrees Celsius). Spread the pears equally in a single layer on a baking dish that has been greased with melted coconut oil. Combine the almond milk, vanilla extract, maple syrup, and coconut oil in a mixing dish. Stir everything together well.

2. In a separate large mixing basin, combine the other ingredients. Stir everything together well. Pour the almond milk mixture over the pears after folding it in the bowl.
3. Preheat your oven to around 350°F and bake the baking dish for 30 mins, or until gently browned and set. Serve right away.

Nutrition: Calories: 479 Fat: 34.9g Protein: 8.8g Carbs: 50.1g

---

9.13 Brown Rice Pilaf with Pistachios and Raisins

Prep Time: 15 mins

Cook Time: 15 mins

Servings: 6

Ingredients:

- 1 tbsp extra-virgin olive oil
- 1 cup chopped onion
- ½ cup shredded carrot
- ½ tsp ground cinnamon
- 1 tsp ground cumin - 2 cups brown rice
- 1¾ cups pure orange juice
- ¼ cup water
- ½ cup shelled pistachios
- 1 cup golden raisins
- ½ cup chopped fresh chives

Directions:

1. Heat the olive oil over medium-high heat in a saucepan until it shimmers. Sauté for 5 mins, or until the onion is transparent.
2. Sauté for 1 min, or until fragrant, with the carrots, cinnamon, and cumin.
3. Combine the brown rice, orange juice, and water in a mixing bowl. Bring the water to a boil. Reduce the heat to medium-low and continue to cook for another 7 mins, or until the liquid has nearly completely evaporated.
4. Sprinkle the rice mixture with pistachios, raisins, and chives in a large serving dish. Serve right away.

Nutrition: Calories: 264 Fat: 7.1g Protein: 5.2g Carbs: 48.9g

---

9.14 Cherry, Apricot, and Pecan Brown Rice Bowl

Prep Time: 15 mins

Cook Time: 1 hour & 5 mins

Servings: 2

Ingredients:

- 2 tbsp olive oil
- 2 green onions, sliced
- ½ cup brown rice
- 1 cup low-sodium chicken stock
- 2 tbsp dried cherries
- 4 dried apricots, chopped
- 2 tbsp pecans, toasted and chopped
- Sea salt and freshly ground pepper, to taste

Directions:

1. Heat the olive oil over medium-high heat in a medium saucepan until it shimmers. Sauté for 1 min, or until the green onions are aromatic.
2. Toss in the rice. Stir everything up well, then pour in the chicken stock. Bring the water to a boil. Reduce the heat to a low setting. Cook, covered, for 50 mins, or until the brown rice is tender.
3. Cook for a further 10 mins, or until the cherries, apricots, and pecans are soft.
4. Fill a big serving basin halfway with them. Using a fork, fluff the mixture. Season with a pinch of salt and freshly ground pepper. Serve right away.

Nutrition: Calories: 451 Fat: 25.9g Protein: 8.2g Carbs: 50.4g

---

9.15 Curry Apple Couscous with Leeks and Pecans

Prep Time: 15 mins

Cook Time: 8 mins

Servings: 4

Ingredients:

- 2 tsp extra-virgin olive oil
- 2 leeks, white parts only, sliced
- 1 apple, diced
- 2 cups cooked couscous
- 2 tbsp curry powder
- ½ cup chopped pecans

Directions:

1. Heat the olive oil on moderate heat in a pan until it shimmers. Sauté for 5 mins, or until the leeks are tender.
2. Cook for 3 mins longer, or until the apple is soft. Combine the couscous and curry powder in a mixing bowl. To blend, stir everything together. Transfer to a large serving dish and stir with the pecans before serving.

Nutrition: Calories: 254 Fat: 11.9g Protein: 5.4g Carbs: 34.3g

9.16 Lebanese Flavor Broken Thin Noodles

Prep Time: 15 mins

Cook Time: 25 mins

Servings: 6

Ingredients:

- 1 tbsp extra-virgin olive oil
- 1 (3-oz / 85-g) cup vermicelli, broken into 1- to 1½-inch pieces
- 3 cups shredded cabbage
- 1 cup brown rice
- 3 cups low-sodium vegetable soup
- ½ cup water
- 2 garlic cloves, mashed
- ¼ tsp sea salt
- 1/8 tsp pepper flakes crushed
- ½ cup coarsely chopped cilantro
- Fresh lemon slices, for serving

Directions:

1. Heat the olive oil over medium-high heat in a saucepan until it shimmers. Sauté for 3 mins, or until the vermicelli is toasted. Sauté for 4 mins, or until the cabbage is soft.
2. Combine the brown rice, vegetable soup, and water in a mixing bowl. Season with salt and red pepper flakes after adding the garlic.
3. Over high heat, bring to a boil. Reduce the heat to a low setting. Cover and continue to cook for another 10 mins. Remove the pan from the heat and set it aside for 5 mins without removing the lid.
4. Serve on a big serving dish with cilantro on top. Serve heated with lemon slices squeezed over it.

Nutrition: Calories: 127 Fat: 3.1g Protein: 4.2g Carbs: 22.9g

9.17 Lemony Farro and Avocado Bowl

Prep Time: 15 mins

Cook Time: 25 mins

Servings: 4

Ingredients:

- 1 tbsp plus 2 tsp extra-virgin olive oil, divided
- ½ medium onion, chopped
- 1 carrot, shredded
- 2 garlic cloves, minced
- 1 (6-oz / 170-g) cup pearled farro
- 2 cups low-sodium vegetable soup
- 2 avocados, peeled, pitted, and sliced
- Zest and juice of 1 small lemon
- ¼ tsp sea salt

Directions:

1. Heat 1 tbsp olive oil in a saucepan over medium-high heat until it shimmers. Sauté for 5 mins, or until the onion is transparent. Sauté for 1 min, or until the carrot and garlic are aromatic.
2. Pour the veggie soup over the farro. Over high heat, bring to a boil. Reduce the heat to a low setting. Cook for 20 mins, or until the farro is al dente, with the lid on.
3. Fold in the avocado slices after transferring the farro to a big serving basin. Drizzle with lemon juice and 2 tbsp olive oil after sprinkling lemon zest and salt. Stir thoroughly to combine and serve right away.

NUTRITION: Calories: 210 Fat: 11.1g Protein: 4.2g Carbs: 27.9g

9.18 Rice and Blueberry Stuffed Sweet Potatoes

Prep Time: 15 mins

Cook Time: 20 mins

Servings: 4

Ingredients:

- 2 cups cooked wild rice
- ½ cup dried blueberries
- ½ cup chopped hazelnuts
- ½ cup shredded Swiss chard
- 1 tsp chopped fresh thyme
- 1 scallion, white and green parts, peeled and thinly sliced
- Sea salt and freshly ground black pepper, to taste
- 4 sweet potatoes, baked in the skin until tender

Directions:

1. Preheat the oven to 400 degrees Fahrenheit (205 degrees Celsius). In a large mixing basin, combine all ingredients except the sweet potatoes. Stir everything together well.
2. Cut the top third of the sweet potato lengthwise and scoop off most flesh. After filling the sweet potato with the wild rice mixture, place it on a prepared baking sheet.

3. Bake for 20 mins or until the sweet potato skin is gently browned in a preheated oven. Serve right away.

Nutrition: Calories: 393 Fat: 7.1g Protein: 10.2g Carbs: 76.9g

9.19 Farro Salad Mix

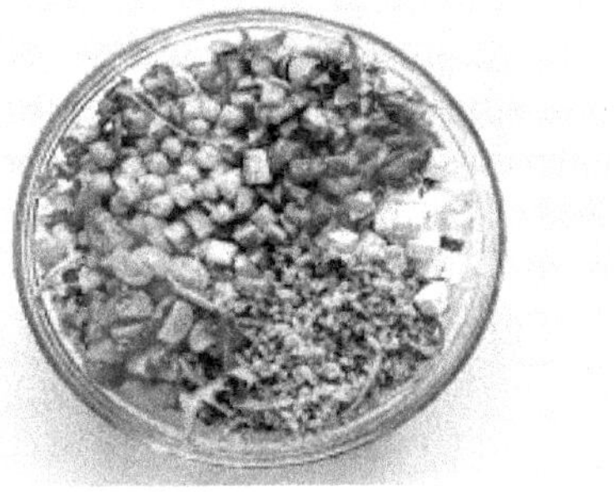

Prep Time: 15 mins

Cook Time: 33 mins

Servings: 4-6

Ingredients:

- 1 tsp Dijon mustard
- 1½ cups whole farro
- 2 oz' feta cheese, crumbled (½ cup)
- 2 tbsp lemon juice
- 2 tbsp minced shallot
- 3 tbsp chopped fresh dill
- 3 tbsp extra-virgin olive oil
- 6 oz' asparagus, trimmed and cut into 1-inch lengths
- 6 oz' cherry tomatoes, halved
- 6 oz' sugar snap peas, strings removed, cut into 1-inch lengths - Salt and pepper

Directions:

1. In a Dutch oven, bring some water to a boil. Cook until the asparagus, snap peas, and 1 tbsp salt are crisp-tender, about 3 mins.
2. Transfer veggies to a large platter with a slotted spoon and set aside to cool fully for approximately 15 mins. Add farro to the boiling water and cook for 15 to 30 mins, or until the grains are soft and chewy.
3. Drain the farro, lay it out on a rimmed baking sheet, and set it aside to cool for 15 mins. In a large mixing bowl, combine the oil, lemon juice, shallot, mustard, 14 tsp salt, and 14 tsp pepper.
4. Toss gently to mix the veggies, farro, tomatoes, dill, and 14 cup feta. Season to taste with salt and pepper. Transfer to a serving plate and top with the remaining 14 cups feta. Serve.

Nutrition: Calories: 240 Carbs: 26g Fat: 12g Protein: 9g

9.20 Farrotto Mix

Prep Time: 15 mins

Cook Time: 40 mins

Servings: 6

Ingredients:

- ½ onion, chopped fine
- 1 cup frozen peas, thawed
- 1 garlic clove, minced
- 1 tbsp minced fresh chives
- 1 tsp grated lemon zest plus 1 tsp juice
- 1½ cups whole farro
- 2 tbsp extra-virgin olive oil
- 2 tsp minced fresh tarragon
- 3 cups chicken broth
- 3 cups water
- 4 oz' asparagus
- 4 oz' pancetta, cut into ¼-inch pieces
- Salt and pepper

Directions:

1. Using a blender, pulse the farro until roughly half of the grains are broken down into smaller pieces, around 6 pulses.
2. In a medium-sized saucepan over high heat, bring broth and water to a boil. Cook for 2 to 3 mins, or until asparagus is crisp-tender.
3. Transfer asparagus to a container with a slotted spoon and set aside. Reduce the heat to low and cover the broth mixture to keep it warm.
4. Cook pancetta in a Dutch oven over medium heat for 5 mins, or until gently browned and fat has rendered.
5. Cook for about 5 mins, until the onion and 1 tbsp of oil have become soft. Add the garlic and simmer for about half a minute, or fragrant.
6. Cook, often turning, until farro grains are gently toasted, about three mins.
7. Stir 5 cups of the heated broth mixture into the farro mixture, reduce the heat to low, cover, and simmer until nearly all the liquid has been absorbed and the farro is just al dente, approximately 25 mins.
8. Cook, constantly stirring, until farro turns creamy, about 5 mins, with peas, tarragon, 34 tsp salt, and 12 tsp pepper.
9. Remove from the fire and stir in the cheese, chives, lemon zest and juice, 1 tbsp oil, and the asparagus set aside.

10. As needed, adjust the consistency with the remaining heated broth mixture (you may have broth left over). Season to taste with salt and pepper. Serve.

Nutrition: Calories: 218 Carbs: 41g Fat: 2g Protein: 7g

9.21 Fennel-thyme Farro

Prep Time: 15 mins

Cook Time: 50 mins

Servings: 4-6

Ingredients:

- ¼ cup minced fresh parsley
- 1 onion, chopped fine - 1 fennel bulb small
- 1 tsp fresh thyme minced
- 1½ cups whole farro
- 2 tsp sherry vinegar
- 3 garlic cloves, minced
- 3 tbsp extra-virgin olive oil
- Salt and pepper

Directions:

1. In a Dutch oven, bring 4 quarts of water to a boil. Return to a boil, add the farro and 1 tbsp salt, & simmer for around 15 to 30 mins, or unless the grains become soft, they have a small crunch.
2. Drain the farro and return it to the now-empty saucepan, covering it to keep it warm. In a 12-inch frying pan, heat 2 tbsp oil over medium heat until it begins to sizzle.
3. Cook, occasionally turning, until the onion, fennel, and 14 tsp salt are soft, 8 to 10 mins. Cook for about half a min until the garlic and thyme are fragrant.
4. Cook, often turning, until the remaining 1 tbsp, oil and farro are cooked through, about 2 mins.
5. Remove the pan from the heat and stir in the parsley and vinegar. Season to taste with salt and pepper. Serve.

Nutrition: Calories: 338 Carbs: 56g Fat: 10g Protein: 11g

9.22 Feta-Grape-Bulgur Salad with Grapes and Feta

Prep Time: 15 mins

Cook Time: 1 hour & 30 mins

Servings: 4-6

Ingredients:

- ¼ cup chopped fresh mint
- ¼ cup extra-virgin olive oil
- ¼ tsp ground cumin
- ½ cup slivered almonds, toasted
- 1 cup water
- 1½ cups rinsed medium-grind bulgur
- 2 oz' feta cheese, crumbled (½ cup)
- 2 scallions, sliced thin
- 5 tbsp lemon juice
- 6 oz seedless red grapes, quartered (1 cup)
- Pinch cayenne pepper
- Salt and pepper

Directions:

1. Combine the bulgur, water, lemon juice, & salt. Cover and let aside at room temperature for approximately 112 hours, or until grains are softened, and liquid is completely absorbed.
2. In a large mixing bowl, combine the remaining 1 tbsp lemon juice, oil, cumin, cayenne, and 14 tsp salt.
3. Gently stir together the bulgur, grapes, 1/3 cup almonds, 1/3 cup feta, scallions, and mint. Season to taste with salt and pepper. Before serving, top with the remaining almonds and feta cheese.

Nutrition: Calories: 500 Carbs: 45g Fat: 14g Protein: 50g

9.23 Greek Style Meaty Bulgur

Prep Time: 15 mins

Cook Time: 30 mins

Servings: 4-6

Ingredients:

- ½ cup jarred roasted red peppers, rinsed, patted dry, and chopped
- 1 bay leaf
- 1 cup medium-grind bulgur, rinsed
- 1 onion, chopped fine
- 1 tbsp chopped fresh dill
- 1 tsp extra-virgin olive oil
- 1 1/3 cups vegetable broth
- 2 tsp minced fresh marjoram or ½ tsp dried
- 3 garlic cloves, minced
- 8 oz ground lamb
- Lemon wedges
- Salt and pepper

Directions:

1. Heat the oil over moderate to high heat in a large saucepan until it just begins to smoke. Add the lamb, 12 tsp salt, and 14 tsp pepper and simmer for 3 to 5 mins,

breaking up the meat with a wooden spoon as it browns.
2. Add the onion and red peppers and simmer for 5 to 7 mins, or until the onion is softened. Cook, constantly stirring, until the garlic and marjoram are fragrant, about half a min.
3. Bring the bulgur, broth, and bay leaf to a boil. Reduce heat to low, cover, and cook for 16 to 18 mins, or until bulgur is soft.
4. Remove the bulgur from the heat, place a clean dish towel beneath the cover, and set aside for 10 mins.
5. Toss in the dill and gently fluff with a fork to mix. Season to taste with salt and pepper. Serve with lemon slices on the side.

Nutrition: Calories: 137 Carbs: 16g Fat: 5g Protein: 7g

9.24 Hearty Barley Mix

Prep Time: 15 mins

Cook Time: 50 mins

Servings: 4

Ingredients:

- 1/8 tsp ground cardamom
- ½ cup plain yogurt
- ½ tsp ground cumin
- 2/3 cup raw sunflower seeds
- ¾ tsp ground coriander
- 1 cup pearl barley
- 1½ tbsp minced fresh mint
- 1½ tsp grated lemon zest plus 1½ tbsp juice
- 3 tbsp extra-virgin olive oil
- 5 carrots, peeled
- 8 oz' snow peas, strings removed, halved along the length
- Salt and pepper

Directions:

1. In a small container, combine yogurt, 12 tsp lemon zest and 112 tsp juice, 112 tsp mint, 14 tsp salt, and 1/8 tsp pepper; cover and chill until ready to serve.
2. In a Dutch oven, bring 4 quarts of water to a boil. Return to a boil, add the barley and 1 tbsp salt, and simmer for 20 to 40 mins, or until cooked. Drain the barley and return it to the now-empty saucepan, covering it to keep it warm.
3. Meanwhile, cut carrots in half crosswise, then halve or quarter them lengthwise to get equally sized pieces.
4. In a 12-inch frying pan, heat 1 tbsp oil over moderate to high heat until it smokes. Cook, occasionally turning, until moderately browned and barely cooked, 5 to 7 mins, with carrots and 12 tsp coriander.
5. Cook, occasionally stirring, until the snow peas are spotty brown, 3 to 5 mins, transfer to a platter.
6. In the now-empty frying pan, heat 112 tbsp oil over medium heat until it begins to shimmer. Sunflower seeds, cumin, cardamom, the remaining 14 tsp coriander, and 14 tsp salt should be added now.
7. Cook, constantly stirring, for about 2 mins, or until seeds are toasted; transfer to a small container.
8. In a large mixing bowl, combine the remaining 1 tsp lemon zest and 1 tbsp juice, 1 tbsp mint, and the remaining 112 tsp oil.
9. Toss the barley and carrot–snow pea combination together carefully. Season with salt and pepper to suit, then serve seasoned sunflower seeds and yogurt sauce drizzled over individual pieces.

Nutrition: Calories: 193 Carbs: 44g Fat: 1g Protein: 4g

9.25 Hearty Barley Risotto

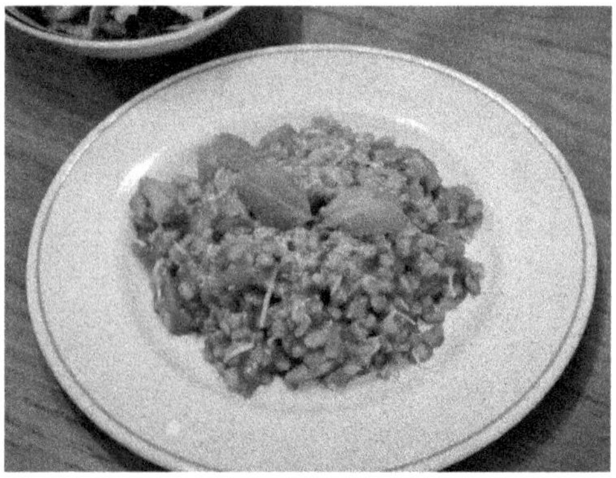

Prep Time: 15 mins

Cook Time: 60 mins

Servings: 4-6

Ingredients:

- 1 carrot, peeled & chopped fine
- 1 cup dry white wine
- 1 onion, chopped fine
- 1 tsp fresh thyme minced
- 1½ cups pearl barley
- 2 tbsp extra-virgin olive oil
- 4 cups of chicken broth
- 4 cups water
- Salt and pepper

Directions:

1. In a medium-sized saucepan, bring broth and water to a simmer. Reduce the heat to a low setting and cover to stay warm.
2. In a Dutch oven, heat 1 tbsp oil over medium heat until it shimmer. Cook, occasionally stirring, until the onion and carrot are soft, about 5 to 7 mins.
3. Cook, turning it regularly until the barley is gently browned and fragrant, approximately 4 mins. Cook, often stirring, until the wine is completely absorbed, about two mins.
4. Add 3 cups of broth and the thyme, bring to a boil, and cook, occasionally stirring, for 22 to 25 mins, or until liquid is absorbed, and the bottom of the pot is dry.
5. Add 2 cups heated broth, bring to a boil, and cook, occasionally stirring, for 15 to 20 mins, or until liquid is absorbed and the bottom of the pot is dry.
6. Continue to boil the risotto, stirring regularly and adding heated stock as needed to keep the pot bottom from drying out for another 15 to 20 mins, or until the barley is cooked through.
7. Remove from thc heat and adjust the consistency as needed with the remaining heated broth. Toss in the cheese and the remaining 1 tbsp oil, then season with salt and pepper to taste. Serve.

Nutrition: Calories: 222 Carbs: 33g Fat: 5g Protein: 6g

CHAPTER 10:

Appetizers And Snacks

10.1 Smoked Salmon Endive Bites Goat Cheese

Prep Time: 15 mins

Cook Time: 0 mins

Servings: 4

Ingredients:

- 1 package goat cheese herbed
- 3 heads endive
- 1 wild salmon smoked package

Directions:

1. Endive leaves should be separated, and the ends chopped off. Toss endive leaves with goat cheese. Over the top of the goat cheese, place fish pieces. Serve.

Nutrition: Calories: 46 Carbs: 1g Fat: 3g Protein: 3g

10.2 Baked tofu

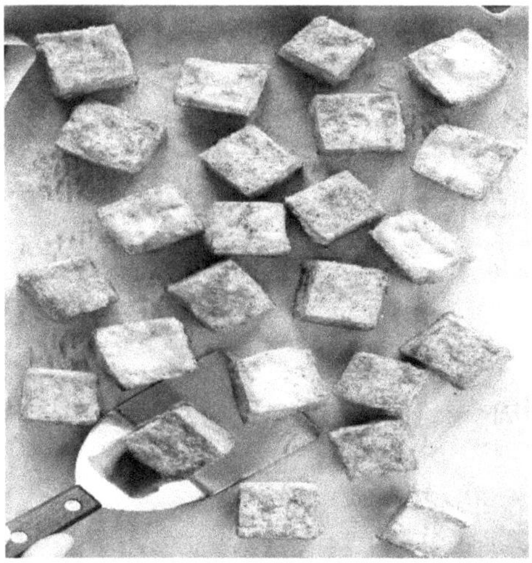

Prep Time: 10 Mins

Cook Time: 10 mins

Servings: 4

Ingredients:

- 250 g Japanese tofu
- 100 g of wheat flour
- 2 tbsp oil
- 100g Daikon radish (Japanese radish)
- 1 piece of fresh ginger
- Japanese soy sauce

Directions:

1. Toss the tofu in cold water for a few seconds.
2. Drain, thoroughly dab and cut into 8 equal cubes with a sharp knife.
3. Toss the tofu pieces in flour and bake in a skillet with heated oil for approximately 1 min on each side, or until golden brown.
4. Peel and coarsely grate the radish and ginger separately. Squeeze the radish and divide it into four equal parts by hand.
5. Place 2 tofu slices on each dish. Place a radish slice next to each and top with ginger and with a dish of Japanese soy sauce on the side.

Nutrition: Calories: 149 Fat: 11.5g Carbs: 8.9g Protein: 2.4g

10.3 Cheesy Cauliflower Frittata

Prep Time: 10 mins

Cook Time: 30 mins

Servings: 4

Ingredients:

- 2 tbsp. olive oil
- 1/2 lb. cauliflower florets
- 1/2 cup skimmed milk
- 6 eggs
- 1 red bell pepper, seeded and chopped
- 1/2 cup Fontina cheese, grated
- 1/2 tsp. red pepper
- 1/2 tsp. turmeric
- Salt and black pepper to taste

Directions

1. Preheat the oven to 360 degrees Fahrenheit. In a mixing dish, whisk together the eggs and milk. Combine the Fontina cheese, red pepper, turmeric, salt, and pepper in a mixing bowl. Add the red bell pepper to the mix. In a pan, heat the olive oil and pour in the egg mixture; cook for 4-5 mins. Remove from the equation.
2. In a saucepan, blanch the cauliflower florets for 5 mins or until tender. Spread the egg mixture on top. Preheat your oven

to around 350°F and bake the skillet for 15 mins, or until golden brown. Allow cooling completely before slicing. Slice and serve.

Nutrition: Calories: 123 Fat: 11 g Carbs: 7 g Protein: 14 g

10.4 Cilantro Mozzarella and Olive Cakes

Prep Time: 10 mins

Cook Time: 25 mins

Servings: 6

Ingredients:

- 1/4 cup black olives
- 1/2 cup low-fat milk
- 4 tbsp. coconut oil softened
- 1 egg, beaten
- 1 cup corn flour
- 1 tsp. baking powder
- 3 sun-dried tomatoes, finely chopped
- 2 tbsp. fresh parsley, chopped
- 2 tbsp. fresh cilantro, chopped
- 1/4 tsp. kosher salt

Directions

1. Preheat the oven to 360 degrees Fahrenheit. Whisk the egg, milk, and coconut oil in a mixing dish. Combine the salt, corn flour, cilantro, and baking powder in a separate basin.
2. Combine the wet and dry ingredients in a mixing bowl. Add the black olives, tomatoes, and herbs and mix well. Bake for 18-20 mins, or until the mixture is done and golden, in buttered ramekins.

Nutrition: Calories: 323 Fat: 11 g Carbs: 6 g Protein: 14.3 g

10.5 Mushroom and Quinoa Cups

Prep Time: 10 mins

Cook Time: 30 mins

Servings: 6

Ingredients:

- 6 eggs
- 1 cup quinoa, cooked
- Salt and black pepper to taste
- 1 cup Gruyere cheese, grated
- 1 small yellow onion, chopped
- 1 cup mushrooms, sliced
- 1/2 cup green olives, chopped

Directions:

1. Whisk the eggs, salt, pepper, Gruyere cheese, onion, mushrooms, and green olives in a mixing bowl.
2. Bake for 30 mins at 360 degrees F on a silicone muffin pan. Warm the dish before serving.

Nutrition: Calories: 233 Fat: 12 g Carbs: 4 g Protein: 21 g

10.6 Zucchini and Mushroom Egg Cakes

Prep Time: 10 mins

Cook Time: 15 mins

Servings: 4

Ingredients:

- 1 onion, chopped
- 1 cup mushrooms, sliced
- 1 red bell pepper, chopped
- 1 zucchini, chopped
- Salt and black pepper to taste
- 8 eggs, whisked
- 1 tbsp. olive oil
- 2 tbsp. chives, chopped

Directions:

1. Preheat the oven to 360 degrees Fahrenheit. In a pan over medium heat, warm the olive oil and cook the onion, zucchini, mushrooms, salt, and pepper for 5 mins, or until soft. Fill muffin cups halfway with the mixture, then top with the eggs.
2. Bake for 10 mins after seasoning with salt, pepper, and chives. Serve right away.

Nutrition: Calories: 245 Fat: 12 g Carbs: 2 g Protein: 12.8 g

10.7 Cinnamon and Coconut Porridge

Prep Time: 5 mins

Cook Time: 5 mins

Servings: 4

Ingredients:

- 1 cup water
- 1/2 cup 36-percent low-fat cream
- 1/2 cup unsweetened dried coconut, shredded
- 1 tbsp oat bran
- 1 tbsp flaxseed meal
- 1/2 tbsp almond butter
- 1 1/2 tsp stevia
- 1/2 tsp cinnamon
- Toppings, such as blueberries or banana slices

Directions:

1. In a small saucepan, combine all ingredients and stir well until well combined. Bring the mixture to a gentle boil in the saucepan on your stove over medium-low heat.
2. Remove from the heat after thoroughly stirring. Allow for 10 mins of resting time after dividing the mixture into equal halves. Enjoy with your preferred toppings!

Nutrition: Calories: 276 Fat: 21 Carbs: 3 g Protein: 13.9g

10.8 Banana Steel Oats

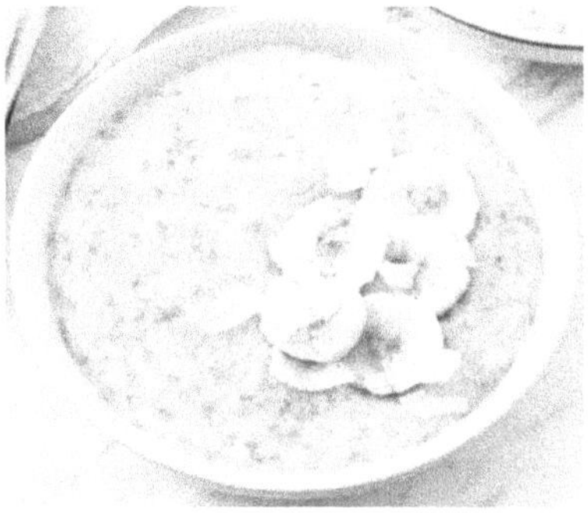

Prep Time: 10 mins

Cook Time: 10 mins

Servings: 3

Ingredients:

- 1 small banana - 1 cup almond milk
- 1/4 tsp cinnamon, ground
- 1/2 cup rolled oats - 1 tbsp honey

Directions:

1. Combine half of the banana, almond milk, and ground cinnamon in a saucepan. Sunflower seeds may be used as a seasoning.
2. Stir until the banana is well mashed, then bring to a boil and add the oats. Reduce to low heat and cook for 5-7 mins, or until the oats are soft. Place the remaining half of the banana on top of the oats and dice it. Enjoy!

Nutrition: Calories: 244 Fat: 11 Carbs: 2 g Protein: 13 g

10.9 Almond Crackers & Crunchy Flax

Prep Time: 20 mins

Cook Time: 60 mins

Servings: 12

Ingredients:

- ½ cup of ground flaxseeds
- ½ cup of almond flour
- 2 tbsp coconut flour
- 2 tbsp shelled hemp seeds
- 1/4 tsp sunflower seeds
- 1 egg white
- 2 tbsp unsalted almond butter, melted

Directions:

1. Preheat the oven to 300 degrees F. Keep a baking pan lined with parchment paper to the side. Combine flax, hemp seed, coconut flour, almond, & seeds. Combine the egg white and melted almond butter in a mixing bowl.
2. Place dough on a parchment paper sheet & cover with a second layer of parchment paper. Prepare the dough by rolling it out. Bake for around 60 mins after cutting into crackers. Allow them to cool before eating.

Nutrition: Calories: 143 Fat: 11 g Carbs: 3 g Protein: 11 g

10.10 Quinoa and Cinnamon Bowl

Prep Time: 10 mins

Cook Time: 15 mins

Servings: 2

Ingredients:

- 1 cup uncooked quinoa
- 11/2 cups water
- 1/2 tsp ground cinnamon
- 1/2 tsp sunflower seeds
- A drizzle of almond/coconut milk for serving

Directions:

1. Quinoa should be well rinsed under water. Add the quinoa, water, cinnamon, and seeds to a medium-sized pot. Place it over medium-high heat and stir it constantly. Bring the ingredients to a boil. Reduce the heat to a low setting and let it simmer.
2. Remove it from the fire and set it aside to cool. Drizzle with almond or coconut milk before serving. Enjoy!

Nutrition: Calories: 165 Fat: 9 g Carbs: 3 g Protein: 9 g

10.11 Quinoa and Date Bowl

Prep Time: 10 mins

Cook Time: 15 mins

Servings: 2

Ingredients:

- 1 date, pitted and chopped finely
- 1/2 cup red quinoa, dried

- 1 cup unsweetened almond milk
- 1/8 tsp vanilla extract
- 1/4 cup fresh strawberries
- 1/8 tsp ground cinnamon

Directions:

1. Place a pan on a low heat setting. Cook for approximately 15 mins, occasionally stirring, after adding the quinoa, almond milk, cinnamon, and vanilla.
2. Serve with strawberries as a garnish.

Nutrition: Calories: 323 Fat: 11 g Carbs: 6 g Protein: 14.3 g

---

10.12 Chickpea Snack Mix

Prep Time: 10 mins

Cook Time: 30 mins

Servings: 8

Ingredients:

- 1 cup roasted chickpeas, drained
- 2 tbsp coconut oil, melted
- 1/4 cup raw pumpkin seeds
- 1/4 cup raw pecan halves
- 1/3 cup dried cherries

Directions

1. Using paper towels, pat the chickpeas dry. Drizzle the chickpeas with coconut oil.
2. Preheat the oven to 380 degrees F and roast the chickpeas for approximately 20 mins, stirring once or twice.
3. Combine the chickpeas, pumpkin seeds, and pecan halves in a mixing bowl. Continue baking for another 8 mins, or until the nuts are aromatic; cool completely.
4. Stir in the dried cherries until everything is well combined. Good appetite!

Nutrition: Calories: 109 Fat: 7.9g Carbs: 7.4g Protein: 3.4g

10.13 Muhammara Dip with a Twist

Prep Time: 10 mins

Cook Time: 35 mins

Servings: 9

Ingredients:

- 3 red bell peppers - 5 tbsp olive oil
- 2 garlic cloves, chopped
- 1 tomato, chopped
- 3/4 cup breadcrumbs
- 2 tbsp molasses
- 1 tsp ground cumin
- 1/4 sunflower seeds, toasted
- 1 Maras pepper, minced - 2 tbsp tahini
- Sea salt and red pepper, to taste

Directions

1. Preheat the oven to 400 degrees Fahrenheit. Place the peppers on a baking sheet lined with parchment paper. After baking for 30 mins, peel the peppers and place them in a food processor.
2. Meanwhile, in a frying pan over medium-high heat, heat 2 tbsp olive oil. Cook for approximately 5 mins, or until the garlic and tomatoes have softened.
3. In a food processor, combine the sautéed veggies. Combine the remaining ingredients in a food processor and pulse until creamy and smooth.
4. Good appetite!

Nutrition: Calories: 149 Fat: 11.5g Carbs: 8.9g Protein: 2.4g

---

10.14 Spinach, Chickpea and Garlic Crostini

Prep Time: 10 mins

Cook Time: 10 mins

Servings: 6

Ingredients:

- 1 baguette, cut into slices
- 4 tbsp extra-virgin olive oil
- Sea salt and red pepper to season
- 3 garlic cloves, minced
- 1 cup boiled chickpeas, drained
- 2 cups spinach - 1 tbsp fresh lemon juice

Directions

1. Preheat the oven to broil.
2. Brush 2 tbsp olive oil over the bread pieces and season with sea salt and red pepper. Place in the broiler for 2 mins or until gently roasted.
3. Combine the garlic, chickpeas, spinach, lemon juice, and the remaining 2 tbsp of olive oil in a mixing bowl.
4. Using a spoon, spread the chickpea mixture on each toast. Good appetite!

Nutrition: Calories: 242 Fat: 6.1g Carbs: 38.5g Protein: 8.9g

---

10.15 Mushroom and Cannellini Bean "Meatballs."

Prep Time: 10 mins

Cook Time: 15 mins

Servings: 4

Ingredients:

- 4 tbsp olive oil

- 1 cup button mushrooms, chopped
- 1 shallot, chopped
- 2 garlic cloves, crushed
- 1 cup canned or boiled cannellini beans, drained
- 1 cup quinoa, cooked
- Sea salt and ground black pepper to flavor
- 1 tsp smoked paprika
- 1/2 tsp red pepper flakes
- 1 tsp mustard seeds
- 1/2 tsp dried dill

Directions

1. In a nonstick skillet, heat 2 tbsp of olive oil. Cook for 3 mins, or until the mushrooms and shallot are barely soft, once the pan is heated.
2. Combine the garlic, beans, quinoa, and spices in a large mixing bowl. Mix well, then roll the mixture into equal balls using lubricated hands.
3. Then, heat the remaining 2 tbsp of olive oil in a nonstick pan over medium heat. Fry the meatballs for approximately 10 mins, or until golden brown on both sides, after the oil is heated.
4. Serve with cocktail sticks on the side. Good appetite!

Nutrition: Calories: 195 Fat: 14.1g Carbs: 13.2g Protein: 3.9g

10.16 Cucumber Rounds with Hummus

Prep Time: 10 mins

Cook Time: 0 mins

Servings: 6

Ingredients:

- 1 cup hummus, preferably homemade
- 2 large tomatoes, diced
- 1/2 tsp red pepper flakes
- Sea salt and ground black pepper to flavor
- 2 English cucumbers, sliced into rounds

Directions

1. Toss the cucumber rounds with the hummus dip.
2. Sprinkle red pepper flakes, salt, and black pepper over each cucumber before serving.
3. Enjoy while it's still cold!

Nutrition: Calories: 88 Fat: 3.6g Carbs: 11.3g Protein: 2.6g

10.17 Stuffed Jalapeño Bites

Prep Time: 10 mins

Cook Time: 15 mins

Servings: 6

Ingredients:

- 1/2 cup raw sunflower seeds, soaked overnight, and drained
- 4 tbsp scallions, chopped
- 1 tsp garlic, minced
- 3 tbsp nutritional yeast
- 1/2 cup cream of onion soup
- 1/2 tsp cayenne pepper
- 1/2 tsp mustard seeds
- 12 jalapeños, halved and seeded
- 1/2 cup breadcrumbs

Directions

1. Blitz raw sunflower seeds, scallions, garlic, nutritional yeast, soup, cayenne pepper, and mustard seeds in a food processor or high-powered blender until fully blended.
2. Fill the jalapenos halfway with the mixture and top with breadcrumbs.
3. Preheat your oven to around 350°F. Warm the dish before serving.

Nutrition: Calories: 108 Fat: 6.6g Carbs: 7.3g Protein: 5.3g

10.18 Mexican-Style Onion Rings

Prep Time: 10 mins

Cook Time: 35 mins

Servings: 6

Ingredients:

- 2 medium onions, cut into rings
- 1/4 cup all-purpose flour
- 1/4 cup spelled flour
- 1/3 cup rice milk, unsweetened
- 1/3 cup ale beer
- Sea salt and ground black pepper to flavor
- 1/2 tsp cayenne pepper
- 1/2 tsp mustard seeds
- 1 cup tortilla chips, crushed
- 1 tbsp olive oil

Directions

1. Preheat the oven to 420 degrees Fahrenheit.
2. Combine the flour, milk, and beer in a small basin.
3. Combine the seasonings and crumbled tortilla chips in a small basin. Toss the onion rings in the flour mixture and set them aside.

4. Then roll them in the spicy mixture, pressing them down to thoroughly coat them.
5. Arrange the onion rings on a baking tray coated with parchment paper. Bake for 30 mins after brushing them with olive oil.

Nutrition: Calories: 213 Fat: 10.6g Carbs: 26.2g Protein: 4.3g

10.19 Roasted Root Vegetables

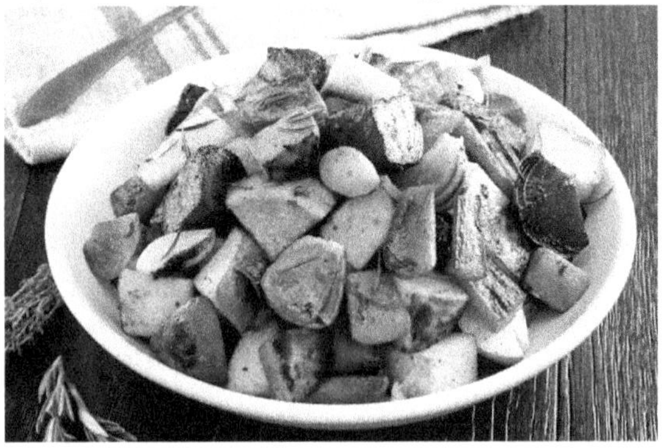

Prep Time: 10 mins

Cook Time: 35 mins

Servings: 6

Ingredients:

- 1/4 cup olive oil
- 2 carrots, peeled and cut
- 2 parsnips, peeled and cut
- 1 celery stalk, peeled and cut
- 1-pound sweet potatoes, peeled and cut
- 1/4 cup olive oil
- 1 tsp mustard seeds
- 1/2 tsp basil
- 1/2 tsp oregano
- 1 tsp red pepper flakes
- 1 tsp dried thyme
- Sea salt and ground black pepper to flavor

Directions

1. Toss the veggies with the other ingredients until they are well distributed.
2. Preheat the oven to 400 degrees F and roast the veggies for 35 mins, stirring halfway during the cooking time.
3. Taste, season with salt and pepper, and serve warm.

Nutrition: Calories: 261 Fat: 18.2g Carbs: 23.3g Protein: 2.3g

10.20 Indian-Style Hummus Dip

Prep Time: 10 mins

Cook Time: 0 mins

Servings: 6

Ingredients:

- 20 oz canned or boiled chickpeas, drained
- 1 tsp garlic, sliced
- 1/4 cup tahini
- 1/4 cup olive oil
- 1 lime, freshly squeezed
- 1/4 tsp turmeric
- 1/2 tsp cumin powder
- 1 tsp curry powder
- 1 tsp coriander seeds
- 1/4 cup chickpea liquid, or more, as needed
- 2 tbsp fresh cilantro, roughly chopped

Directions

1. In a blender or food processor, combine the chickpeas, garlic, tahini, olive oil, lime, turmeric, cumin, curry powder, and coriander seeds.
2. Blend until you have the appropriate consistency, then slowly drizzle in the chickpea liquid.
3. Put it in the fridge until you're ready to serve. Serve with fresh cilantro as a garnish.
4. If preferred, serve with naan bread or vegetable sticks.

Nutrition: Calories: 171 Fat: 10.4g Carbs: 15.3g Protein: 5.4g

CHAPTER 11:

Snack & Dessert

11.1 Nacho Cheese

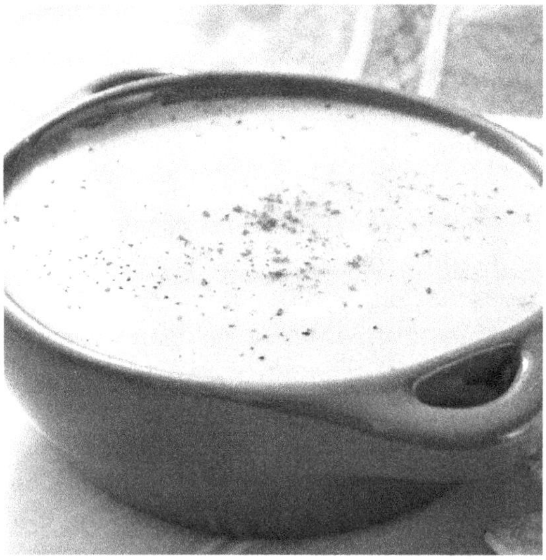

Prep Time: 10 mins
Cook Time: 15 mins
Servings: 4
Ingredients:

- 2 cups peeled chopped russet potatoes
- 1 cup chopped carrots
- 1/2 to 3/4 cup water
- 1 tbsp freshly squeezed lemon juice
- 1/2 cup nutritional yeast
- 1/2 tsp onion powder
- 1/2 tsp garlic powder
- 1 tsp salt
- 1/4 cup Super-Simple Salsa (here) or store-bought (optional)

Directions:

1. Cook the potatoes and carrots for approximately 15 mins, or until they are tender.
2. In a blender, combine 1/2 cup water, lemon juice, nutritional yeast, onion powder, garlic powder, salt, and salsa (if using). Blend until the mixture is smooth. If the consistency is too thick, thin it out with the remaining 1/4 cup of water.

Nutrition: Calories: 237 Fat: 1g Protein: 13g Carbs: 24g

11.2 Mushroom Gravy

Prep Time: 10 mins
Cook Time: 10 mins
Servings: 4
Ingredients:

- 1 tbsp oil
- 1 small yellow onion, diced
- 1 cup finely chopped button mushrooms
- 11/2 tsp minced garlic (3 cloves)
- 4 tbsp flour
- 11/4 cups water
- 1 tbsp soy sauce
- 1/2 tsp dried oregano
- 2 bay leaves
- Freshly ground black pepper

Directions:

1. In a saucepan, heat the oil, then add the onion, mushrooms, and garlic. Sauté the onions until they are transparent.
2. Mix in the flour until a thick mixture forms.
3. Over medium heat, bring the water, soy sauce, oregano, and bay leaves to a simmer. Season with salt and pepper.
4. Remove the bay leaves from the dish. Gently combine the gravy with a whisk until it thickens. If you like a thinner gravy, add extra water.

Nutrition: Calories: 79 Fat: 4g Protein: 2g Carbs: 9g

11.3 The Greatest Guacamole

Prep Time: 10 mins
Cook Time: 0 mins
Servings: 4
Ingredients:

- 2 large avocados, halved, peeled, and roughly chopped
- Juice of 1/2 lime
- 2 tsp olive oil
- 1/4 red onion, finely diced
- 1/2 tsp minced garlic (1 clove)
- 1/2 tsp ground cumin

- 1 tbsp freshly chopped cilantro
- 1/2 Roma tomato, diced
- Pinch salt
- Freshly ground black pepper

Directions:

1. In a medium-sized mixing bowl, mash the avocados to desired consistency.
2. Combine the lime juice and oil in a mixing bowl. Season with salt and pepper after adding the red onion, garlic, cumin, cilantro, and tomato.

Nutrition: Calories: 233 Fat: 22g Protein: 2g Carbs: 9g

11.4 Super Simple Salsa

Prep Time: 10 mins

Cook Time: 0 mins

Servings: 4

Ingredients:

- 2 cups chopped tomatoes
- 1/2 cup diced yellow onion
- 2 tbsp minced cilantro
- Juice of 1/2 lime, plus more for seasoning (optional)
- 1 jalapeño pepper, seeded and chopped
- 1/2 tsp ground cumin
- Pinch salt
- Freshly ground black pepper

Directions:

1. Combine the tomatoes, onion, cilantro, lime juice, jalapeno, and cumin in a mixing bowl.
2. Season with salt and pepper, then squeeze in extra lime juice if desired (if using).

Nutrition: Calories: 25 Fat: 1g Protein: 1g Carbs: 14g

11.5 Cashew Cream

Prep Time: 5 mins

Cook Time: 0 mins

Servings: 4

Ingredients:

- 1 cup raw cashews,
- 1/2 cup water - 1/4 tsp salt
- Freshly ground black pepper

Directions:

1. In a high-powered blender or food processor, combine the soaked cashews, water, and salt, mix until smooth.
2. Season with salt and pepper.

Nutrition: Calories: 197 Fat: 16g Protein: 5g Carbs: 8g

11.6 Spinach Dip

Prep Time: 20 Mins

Cook Time: 5 Mins

Servings: 8

Ingredients:

- ¾ cup cashews
- 3.5 oz' soft tofu
- 6 oz of spinach leaves
- 1 medium white onion, peeled, diced
- 2 tsp minced garlic
- ½ tsp salt
- 3 tbsp olive oil

Directions:

1. In a dish, place the cashews, cover with boiling water, and soak for 15 mins.
2. Drain the cashews after 15 mins and put them aside until needed.
3. Place a medium skillet pan over medium heat, add oil, and remove the pan from the heat.
4. Add the onion and sauté for 3 to 5 mins, or until soft. Stir in the garlic and simmer for another 30 seconds, or until fragrant.
5. Fill a blender halfway with the onion mixture, add the additional ingredients, and whirl until smooth.
6. Serve with chips after transferring the dip to a bowl.

Nutrition: Calories: 134.6 Fat: 8.6 g Protein: 10 g Carbs: 6.3 g

11.7 Tomatillo Salsa

Prep Time: 5 Mins

Cook Time: 15 Mins

Servings: 8

Ingredients:

- 5 medium tomatillos, chopped
- 3 cloves of garlic, peeled, chopped
- 3 Roma tomatoes, chopped
- 1 jalapeno, chopped
- ½ of a medium red onion, peeled, chopped
- 1 Anaheim chili
- 2 tsp salt
- 1 tsp ground cumin
- 1 lime, juiced
- ¼ cup cilantro leaves
- ¾ cup of water

Directions:

1. Pour water into a medium saucepan over medium heat, then add the onion,

tomatoes, tomatillo, jalapeño, and Anaheim chili.
2. After 15 mins of cooking, take the pot from the heat, add the cilantro and lime juice, and season with salt. Remove the saucepan from the heat and mix until smooth with an immersion blender.
3. With chips, serve the salsa.

Nutrition: Calories: 317.4 Fat: 0 g Protein: 16 g Carbs: 64 g

11.8 Arugula Pesto Couscous

Prep Time: 10 Mins

Cook Time: 20 Mins

Servings: 4

Ingredients:

- 8 oz' Israeli couscous
- 3 large tomatoes, chopped
- 3 cups arugula leaves
- ½ cup parsley leaves
- 6 cloves of garlic, peeled
- ½ cup walnuts - ¾ tsp salt
- 1 cup and 1 tbsp olive oil
- 2 cups vegetable broth

Directions:

1. Place 1 tbsp oil in a medium saucepan over medium-high heat and let to heat.
2. Cook for 4 mins, constantly stirring, until couscous is aromatic and toasted.
3. Pour in the broth, swirl to combine, bring to a boil, reduce to low heat, and continue to cook for 12 mins, or until the couscous has absorbed all the liquid and is soft.
4. Remove the pan from the heat, fluff it up with a fork, and leave it aside until needed.
5. Prepare the pesto while the couscous is cooking. To do so, pour walnuts into a blender, add garlic, and process until the nuts have broken down. Pulse in the arugula, parsley, and salt until thoroughly incorporated, then add the oil & blend unless smooth. Toss the couscous with the tomatoes and pesto in a salad bowl until well combined. Serve immediately.

Nutrition: Calories: 73 Fat: 4 g Protein: 2 g Carbs: 8 g

11.9 Pico de Gallo

Prep Time: 5 Mins

Cook Time: 0 Mins

Servings: 6

Ingredients:

- ½ of a medium red onion, peeled, chopped
- 2 cups diced tomato
- ½ cup chopped cilantro
- 1 jalapeno pepper, minced
- 1/8 tsp salt
- ¼ tsp ground black pepper
- ½ of a lime, juiced
- 1 tsp olive oil

Directions:

1. Place all ingredients in a large mixing basin and toss until thoroughly combined.
2. With chips, serve the Pico de Gallo.

Nutrition: Calories: 790 Fat: 6.4 g Protein: 25.6 g Carbs: 195.2 g

11.10 Beet Balls

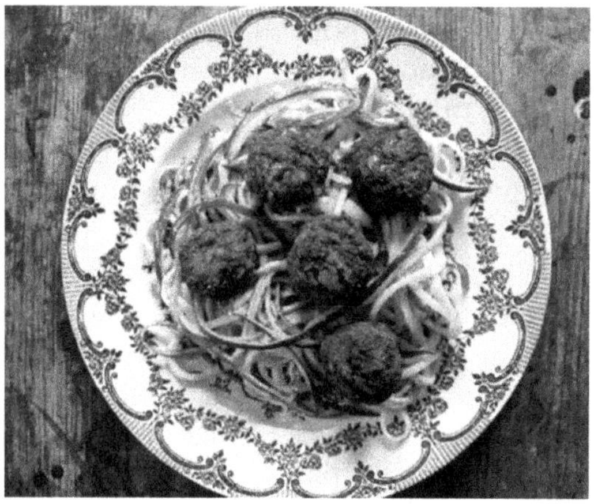

Prep Time: 10 Mins

Cook Time: 0 Mins

Servings: 6

Ingredients:

- ½ cup oats
- 1 medium beet, cooked
- ½ cup almond flour
- 1/3 cup shredded coconut and more for coating
- ¾ cup Medjool dates pitted
- 1 tbsp cocoa powder
- ¼ cup chocolate chips, unsweetened

Directions:

1. Place cooked beets in a blender and pulse until they are finely minced.
2. Pulse in the remaining ingredients until the dough comes together.
3. Form the dough into eighteen balls, then roll them in additional coconut before serving.

Nutrition: Calories: 114.2 Fat: 2.4 g Protein: 5 g Carbs: 19.6 g

11.11 Cheesy Crackers

Prep Time: 10 Mins

Cook Time: 20 Mins

Servings: 3

Ingredients:

- 1 ¾ cup almond meal
- 3 tbsp nutritional yeast
- ½ tsp of sea salt
- 2 tbsp lemon juice
- 1 tbsp melted coconut oil
- 1 tbsp ground flaxseed
- 2 ½ tbsp water

Directions:

1. Preheat your oven to around 350 degrees Fahrenheit after turning it on.
2. Meanwhile, pour flaxseed in a medium mixing bowl, whisk in water, and set aside for 5 mins until thickened.
3. In a medium mixing basin, combine almond meal, salt, yeast, and whisk until well combined.
4. Whisk the flaxseed mixture with the lemon juice and oil until well combined.
5. Pour the flaxseed mixture into the almond meal mixture and stir until the dough forms. Set a piece of wax paper on a clean work surface, place the dough on top of it, cover with another piece of wax paper, and roll the dough into a 1/8-inch-thick crust.
6. Cut the dough into a square, season with salt, and bake for 15 to 20 mins, or until done. Serve immediately.

Nutrition: Calories: 30 Fat: 1 g Protein: 1 g Carbs: 5 g

11.12 Tomato Soup

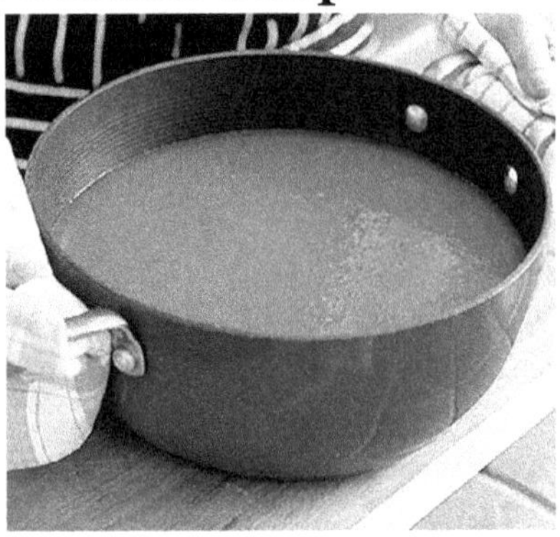

Prep Time: 10 Mins

Cook Time: 10 Mins

Servings: 2

Ingredients:

- 56 oz stewed tomatoes
- ¼ tsp salt
- ¼ tsp ground black pepper
- 1 medium red bell pepper, cored, diced
- ¼ tsp dried thyme
- 6 leaves of basil, chopped
- ¼ tsp dried oregano
- 1 tsp olive oil

Directions:

1. Place a medium saucepan over medium heat, add the oil, add the bell pepper, and cook for 4 minutes after it's heated.
2. Add the other ingredients to the saucepan, whisk to combine, then reduce heat to medium-high and bring to a boil.
3. Remove the soup from the heat and purée until smooth.
4. Season with salt & pepper to taste, then spoon soup into bowls and serve.

Nutrition: Calories: 170 Fat: 1.1 g Protein: 3.5 g Carbs: 36 g

11.13 Meatballs Platter

Prep Time: 10 Mins

Cook Time: 15 Mins

Servings: 4

Ingredients:

- 1-pound beef meat, ground
- ¼ cup panko breadcrumbs
- A pinch of salt and black pepper
- 3 tbsp red onion, grated
- ¼ cup parsley, chopped
- 2 garlic cloves, minced
- 2 tbsp lemon juice
- Zest of 1 lemon, grated
- 1 egg
- ½ tsp cumin, ground
- ½ tsp coriander, ground
- ¼ tsp cinnamon powder
- 2 oz feta cheese, crumbled
- Cooking spray

Directions:

1. In a mixing bowl, combine the meat, breadcrumbs, salt, pepper, and the other ingredients (excluding the cooking spray), toss well, and roll into medium balls.
2. Place the meatballs on a parchment-lined baking sheet, coat with cooking spray, and bake for 15 mins at 450 degrees F.
3. Serve the meatballs as a snack by placing them on a dish.

Nutrition: Calories: 300 Fat: 15.4g Carbs: 22.4g Protein: 35g

11.14 Yogurt Dip

Prep Time: 10 Mins
Cook Time: 0 Mins
Servings: 6

Ingredients:

- 2 cups Greek yogurt
- 2 tbsp pistachios, toasted and chopped
- A pinch of salt and white pepper
- 2 tbsp mint, chopped
- 1 tbsp kalamata olives, pitted and chopped
- ¼ cup za'atar spice
- ¼ cup pomegranate seeds
- 1/3 cup olive oil

Directions:

1. In a mixing bowl, whisk together the yogurt, pistachios, and the other ingredients.
2. Serve with pita chips on the side and divide into tiny cups.

Nutrition: Calories: 294 Fat: 18g Carbs: 21g Protein: 10g

11.15Tomato Bruschetta

Prep Time: 10 Mins
Cook Time: 10 Mins
Servings: 6

Ingredients:

- 1 baguette, sliced
- 1/3 cup basil, chopped
- 6 tomatoes, cubed
- 2 garlic cloves, minced
- A pinch of salt and black pepper
- 1 tsp olive oil
- 1 tbsp balsamic vinegar
- ½ tsp garlic powder
- Cooking spray

Directions:

1. Arrange the baguette slices on a parchment-lined baking sheet, coat with cooking spray, and bake for 10 mins at 400 degrees F.
2. Combine the tomatoes, basil, and additional ingredients in a mixing dish, combine well and set aside for 10 mins.
3. Serve by dividing the tomato mixture among the baguette slices and arranging them on a dish.

Nutrition: Calories: 162 Fat: 4g Carbs: 29g Protein: 4g

Conclusion

The Pegan diet combines the finest elements of both the Paleo and Vegan diets. Dr. Mark Hyman, a family doctor, and head of the Cleveland Clinic's Centre for Functional Medicine promotes the Pegan diet. The Pegan diet is a new fad diet that blends veganism with the paleo diet. The Pegan diet calls for you to cut out all meat and animal products from your diet while increasing your intake of vegetables and plants.

The vegan diet has several benefits, including lowering the risk of obesity, some malignancies, and type 2 diabetes. However, some amino acids, which are the building blocks of protein and can only be obtained via nutrition, lack the diet. It also lacks iron, calcium, zinc, and vitamin B12.

A proper Paleo diet may be too taxing and costly for some people. When you consider the health implications, it's also a concern. On the other hand, veganism is similarly stringent and difficult for individuals to follow. As a result of integrating these two opposed diets, the Pegan diet, which offers a perfect balance of health benefits and few restrictions, makes a lot of sense for those who want to live a healthy lifestyle while agreeing to consume a limited amount of animal-based protein.

Processed foods, such as sodas and grains in prepared dishes, such as bread and other baked products, should be avoided. These toxins are just not good for your body in any manner! You should eat entire foods from all areas of the plant world, such as vegetables, fruits, nuts, seeds, and unsaturated oils (such as olive oil) rather than refined oils since unsaturated oils are better for your heart (e.g., fry oil). Also, stay away from anything fried!

The time it takes to prepare the dish may be improved. It forces you to think about the food before cooking and be patient while doing so. You may relax while you're cooking it, and at the end of it, you'll have a portion of delicious cuisine to share with others. There will be no squandered meals.

You will cook well if you follow the instructions, and your meal will be tastier and of better quality. Some dishes are both enjoyable and healthful. Make your supper more special by creating a unique dish on your own. There will be no other recipes that can create the same stuff as yours in this situation. You may produce a variety of tastes and foods that you can consume.

Simple directions provide further information about the components, and vegan cooking requires patience. The recipe's instructions are nicely stated, and if you want to make superior cuisine, you may carefully follow them.

One of the essential methods to prepare a decent recipe is to take the time to be patient when preparing a piece of tasty cuisine. You must follow the steps outlined in the recipe below. Follow the formula for greater health to live a healthy life.

CPSIA information can be obtained
at www.ICGtesting.com
Printed in the USA
LVHW060051060222
710368LV00013B/339

9 781914 102691